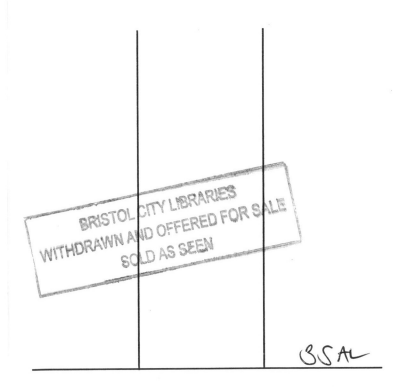
Please return/renew this item by the last date shown
on this label, or on your self-service receipt.

To renew this item, visit **www.librarieswest.org.uk**
or contact your library.

Your Borrower number and PIN are required.

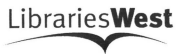

LibrariesWest

D0235016

4 1 0277504 8

Just Like Life, Only More So
and Other Stories of Illness

Dana Snyder-Grant

Library of Congress Control Number: 2006904822

Printed in the United States of America
Trail's End Publishers, Acton, Massachusetts
For ordering information: JustLikeLifeOnlyMoreSo.com

Many of the essays in this book originated in "Connections," the author's column in *The Beacon* (Community Newspaper Company, Concord, Massachusetts), a community newspaper of Acton and Boxborough, Massachusetts.

Additional essays in this book first appeared in the following publications:

AMC Outdoors (May 2000). *The Boston Sunday Globe* (March 4, 2001). *Communities Journal of Cooperative Living* (Spring 1999). *Inside MS* (Summer 2001 and April - June 2004). *KnitLit (too)* (edited by Linda Roghaar and Molly Wolf, Three Rivers Press, 2004). *Real Living with MS* (February 1996). *Reinventing Community: Stories from the Walkways of Cohousing* (edited by Dave Wann, Fulcrum Publishing, 2005).

Cover Design by Julie Sartain

This book is dedicated to the 2.5 million people around the world who have multiple sclerosis.

We tell stories because we can't help it. We tell stories because they save us.

— James Carroll, "The Communion of Sinners"

CONTENTS

Acknowledgments

Thank you to my family for always being there.
Thank you to my clients for letting me witness your stories.
Thank you to my community of friends and neighbors for showing me the deep meanings in connection.
Thank you, RC, for walking this road with me.
And thank you, Jim, for your smile, your patience, and your love.

This book would not have become a reality without all of you.

Introduction

When I woke up on December 1, 1981, my world was spinning. The walls and ceiling moved like a merry-go-round; when I sat up in bed and looked at the apartment building across the street, I saw windows jumping. Any movement of my body, however slight, left me feeling nauseated and dizzy.... I inched slowly along the wall of my apartment to go to the bathroom and then returned to bed. Shattered by the loss of security in my orientation to the world, it was only when I lay down with my eyes closed that I felt safe. But I was scared...this was not like the pins and needles sensations that had taken over the left side of my body for a few weeks in September. That had been scary but mostly it had been annoying. Now I felt horribly ill and...I couldn't see.

— "Red-Letter Day"

One week later, I was diagnosed with multiple sclerosis. It's been twenty-five years since that day.

Living with illness is about living with vulnerability, about being susceptible to loss and hurt. It's just like life, only more so. For we all have vulnerabilities. Your friends earn more money than you do, you have a weight problem, you divorce, you lose your job, a loved one dies. My stories of illness can be generalized to other stories of living. We are all susceptible to loss, all the time, to the losses that come with being human.

I don't mean to say that it's all the same, that living with the unpredictability and disorganization of serious illness is just like other losses. We live in a different world, those of us with unpredictable bodies, deformed bodies, ungainly shuffles. We are more at risk of infirmity and early death. We are stared at, left out, underemployed. But my stories can apply to your life even if you don't live with illness; they can mean something to you.

Please don't withdraw from me out of pity or fear. I want us to stay connected. My story isn't so different from yours. When I am dismayed at myself because I have no balance and use a walker, you judge yourself for not being smart enough or good-looking enough. When I must give up knitting because I no longer have hand coordination, you give up tennis because you have bad knees. When I feel insecure because I am unable to work at a job for many hours, you lose your job during a recession. When I rest instead of attend the party, you work late and miss the festivities. We both have a choice here. You can't determine your work load, but you can control how you manage it. I can't control my illness, but I can control how I respond to it. Illness can make me vulnerable, but your exposure in the world can hurt just as much.

When we're vulnerable, the illusion that we are safe is shattered. It may be a cliché, but vulnerability teaches. It teaches me to appreciate the moment, to value human connection, to cherish the ease of simplicity. I tell my tale to make sense of my illness.

I wrote these essays over the last ten years, many as newspaper columns, to explore issues and events along the way. While editing the essays to create this book, I discovered that I kept returning to a few central themes. So I've organized the book into chapters for each theme, such as the medical journey, loss and change, cultural bias, letting go, nature, and community. But most of the essays address multiple themes. For example, when I write about cultural bias and stigma, I'm often also writing about coping with the loss of physical functioning, hopes, and dreams, all influenced by my own and society's expectations. And in the process, I'm writing about letting go.

The theme of community surfaces throughout my stories. For more than ten years, my husband, Jim, and I have lived in the New View cohousing community in Acton, Massachusetts, with two dozen other families who know and care about each other. My neighbors don't hold the cure for my immune system gone awry, but they provide the support and connection that form my lifeblood, whether I am ill or well.

In various essays, I touch upon my work as a clinical social worker specializing in chronic illness and disability. That work is part of my regeneration, a way to create meaning from what I've been dealt. I devote my final chapter, "Portraits," to a client's story and to the tales of others in my life who have faced illness.

I have dated each essay to indicate when it was written, but I have not put them in a strictly chronological order. This is because the illness journey is not a linear process, but a cyclical one. Grief, accompanied by anger, despair, and acceptance, has always traveled near me, stopping by when I least expect a visitor.

I'm driven to make sense from the MS. Maybe because I've been spared the worst, I want to give back to the world. As a psychotherapist, I bear witness to the stories of others. As a person with MS, I write and speak about illness to discover its meaning. Come with me on my journey.

THE MEDICAL JOURNEY

Red-Letter Day
December 1995

I would have circled the date on my calendar in red pen, December 1, 1981, if I had known its significance in my life. I was one week shy of my twenty-sixth birthday when I was diagnosed with multiple sclerosis. Some of my memories from that week are blurry; others are as clear as if it were yesterday. But I have since come to know with certainty just how much the care of friends and the attention of physicians matters.

It was the Monday after Thanksgiving in 1981. I had just returned from a good visit home with my family. I had felt more separate from my siblings and parents this time. For a little while, I had not been the baby, wondering what they all thought of me, but a more centered adult. That Monday afternoon, after teaching high school, I offered to drive a van of commuting students to the train station. As I exited off the highway, I noticed that my vision was blurry. Something was not quite right. It must have been because I was tired after the long weekend.

I returned to school with the van. My new boyfriend, Kurt, was waiting for me, after coaching the varsity basketball team. We drove to his apartment in Somerville and decided to have dinner together. I lay on his living room floor while he went out for a run, noting that I felt unusually tired. We ate at a gourmet pizza restaurant near my apartment in Cambridge. I spoke little. I was unconcerned about Kurt's thoughts. Both were rare occurrences. We parted company. I prepared little for the next day's lessons, also unusual, and went to bed.

When I woke up the next morning, the world was spinning. The walls and ceiling moved like a merry-go-round; when I sat up in bed and looked at the apartment building across the street, I saw windows jumping. Any movement of my body, however slight, left me feeling nauseated and dizzy. The bedroom in my small Central Square apartment was just across from a tiny kitchen; the bathroom was another small space around a corner. I inched slowly along the wall to go to the bathroom and then returned to bed. Shattered by the loss of security in my orientation to the world, it was only when I lay down with my eyes closed that I felt safe. But I was scared. I had to call in sick. There was no question about going to work. This was not like the pins and needles sensations that had taken over the left side of my body for a few weeks in September. That had been scary but mostly it had been annoying. Now I felt horribly ill and, for all intents and purposes, I couldn't see. The phone was next to the bed; I reached out for it with my right arm, without turning my head, and called the school.

I then phoned my internist, Dr. Nary. I described my symptoms; he guessed that I had an inner ear infection and prescribed some antibiotics, telling me to call again in a day or two if things hadn't cleared up. I hung up the phone, feeling relieved at having communicated my concern to the doctor and satisfied that he would take care of me. We shared a history together, and I still held on to the belief in the all-powerful physician.

I slept most of that day, and it didn't take long to discover that if I covered my left eye, the spinning lessened. So I could lie on my left side in bed and watch the television perched on the desk with my right eye, my left eye closed and resting against the pillow. I must have spoken to Kurt sometime during the day because he dropped off the prescription that afternoon.

Two days later, the dizziness was still present, though less intense. I spoke to Dr. Nary again and reported that I could cover my left eye to relieve the spinning. The immediacy of his response, "I think I should see you tomorrow," took me aback. I heard a concern in his voice that went beyond the caring I had come to know. Perhaps this was something serious. What did these weird sensations of the last few months mean? First the pins and needles, and now the visual distortions. Was I nuts or just stressed? Perhaps the intensity of the class I was teaching on the Holocaust was taking its toll on my psyche. Well, my doctor would take care of it, I again thought. I don't think I could formulate the fear of a brain tumor while I was all alone in my apartment. That would have to wait until the next day.

I called my friends Alan and Sarah, who lived in Watertown near the health center, and asked if I could sleep over and get a ride to my nine o'clock appointment. They readily agreed and Alan came to pick me up. The advantage of having a friend in graduate school, still working on his dissertation, was a flexible schedule. I wouldn't tease Alan anymore about his continuing student status.

Alan had fashioned a makeshift eye patch for me, with gauze to cover the eye and elastic attached to secure the patch around my head. He and Sarah cooked one of their signature Chinese dishes of chicken and water chestnuts. We watched television together. I needed the distraction, which took me out of myself. Nothing was really wrong with me or my body.

In Dr. Nary's office the next day, I was alone in the examining room for some time. Enough time for me to notice that I was trembling with anxiety. The dizziness still lingered. It was serious enough for a doctor to see me on almost immediate notice. Did he think I had a brain tumor? I had the first of many neurological exams. This one focused on my eyes, with Dr. Nary moving his fingers back and forth, up and down. I would cover one eye, then the other. It was clear to both of us that the left eye was the culprit. When it was open, I saw double of everything — four hands, two faces, and more tables than there were in the room. He didn't say much, leaving me with my fears as he left the office. Where the hell was he going?

I began to cry silently. I felt so alone, abandoned by my doctor for a moment, by my body for too long. When he returned, his presence turned those tears into sobs. "What is wrong, Dr. Nary?" I cried. "What is happening?" He then looked at me and said, "Look, I know you are a bright young woman who is probably thinking terrible thoughts." He paused and stared out the door of the examination room. His gaze returned to me as he said, "I don't usually do this, but I will tell you that this could be multiple sclerosis." Although I didn't know what those words meant, their shock numbed my tears. Did this mean that I was going to die? Dr. Nary didn't explain MS to me, but he did the unheard of. He got on the phone to the health center's affiliate hospital and made an appointment for me at one o'clock that afternoon with a neurologist. Maybe doctors can get that kind of response from one another; I now know that patients cannot.

Dr. Marie Fleming was a large, bustling woman. Others who knew her have described her as a drill sergeant, but her direct manner eased my anxiety. She wanted to hear my story. I told her the symptoms of the last few months — the tingling and numbness of September, the double vision of the last week, which was all but cleared up by now. I felt calm as I told my story. The doctor's witness of my testimony offered me a validation and a presence. My story mattered. How much I appreciate this, knowing what I now do of the experience of MS patients who lack a diagnosis for years and only gain referrals to psychiatrists. Or who are told that they have MS, "but there is nothing I can do for you."

After hearing my tale, Dr. Fleming said, "I know exactly what you have. You have multiple sclerosis." My fear and shock returned — this was the stuff of telethons and of other people — but I was blessed by the fact that she let me stay in her office for an hour while I cried and asked questions about the illness. How could this happen to me? I kept thinking she must have a busy schedule, she should kick me out, but instead she patiently answered my torrent of questions. Would I die? Should I move to a different climate? Would the double vision return? What was the difference between multiple sclerosis and muscular dystrophy? I doubt such attention could be given in today's world of managed care.

But on that day, I learned that MS was not fatal nor was it contagious. It was unpredictable. My vision could be impaired but it would likely be temporary. It was unknown if and how my legs or walking would be affected. I learned that for many people with MS, the illness was invisible; symptoms would come and go for years, but I could live a healthy, productive life. I don't think she told me about the worst-case scenarios — the blindness, the wheelchairs. At least that's not what I remember from that day.

What I do remember is deep gratitude for friends who remained present and doctors who attended to my story. I have always felt that my swift diagnosis and my neurologist's quiet understanding of my emotional world contributed to my ability to incorporate this illness into my life. I didn't experience years of doubt from doctors that would make me question my perceptions. My body and my story had been respected. Not that it didn't take years of frequent MS exacerbations to help me adjust to its reality, but I now know the power of being heard as one journeys through our random universe.

Nine days later, my friends and I crowded into my small Cambridge apartment to celebrate my birthday. My brother and sister surprised me, arriving from New York City and Philadelphia for the event. There was a lot of love in that small space.

Dr. Nary later told me that he would have bet his paycheck on my having MS when he saw me on that day of diagnosis, the one that I never did circle on the calendar. He made the decision to call Dr. Fleming and relay the urgency of the referral, because he knew that she specialized in MS. It was some time later that I received a copy of his notes from that fall. In September, Dr. Nary had written about the numbness and tingling, "cannot rule out diagnosis of M.S., etc., but will watch." Then, on the December day when I called him to report dizziness, he wrote, "still worry about M.S." It brings chills to my spine whenever I read these notes, even now, twenty-five years later. I guess that someplace in my memory, that day *is* circled in red.

The Two Neurologists
October 1995

In August, after my husband and I moved to the western suburbs, I had an appointment with Dr. Steven Kelly. He was the doctor recommended by my previous neurologist in Boston. Never mind that his name wasn't the one that everyone else gave me; my doctor's recommendation seemed most important.

I was sad to leave Dr. Lathi's care; she had taken over when my first neurologist, Dr. Fleming, retired, and I had grown to trust her. But I knew it was important that I live near my neurologist. When MS fatigue and more disturbing symptoms intruded into my life, the last thing I wanted was a long drive to see the doctor.

Dr. Kelly, a tall, imposing figure, came into the waiting room. In his office, he asked about the MS. I told him my fourteen-year history, from the horrible early years of severe fatigue, balance loss, and distorted vision to the relative stability of the last five years.

"Did you ever have a spinal tap?" Dr. Kelly asked, rustling the notes that Dr. Lathi had sent him.

"No," I responded. "My neurologist back then was certain my symptoms indicated MS, and she knew a spinal tap would only be painful."

"How about an MRI?" he asked, referring to the more current and accurate diagnostic test for MS.

"No," I again responded, feeling abashed.

"It's unusual to be diagnosed without such confirmation," he replied.

I can't even remember the exam Dr. Kelly gave me. He probably tested my reflexes, assessed my balance and walking. I do know that he did not attend to my weary eyes. Back in his office after the exam, he abruptly said, "I could not tell you had MS, except from your history." Did he mean that as a compliment? Or as a criticism? I imagined the latter. But didn't my story capture the mystery of the hidden symptoms of MS?

Had this doctor heard me when I described my fatigue, my visual disturbances, my troubling sensory symptoms? The heavy arms and legs? The loss of coordination? These intrusive symptoms challenged my life. Worst of all, Dr. Kelly didn't ask about me, who I was, my work, or my family. He reviewed his procedure with new patients. He recommended an MRI and tests to rule out AIDS and Lyme disease, as they could mimic MS. Didn't he believe I had MS? Were the last fourteen years a mirage? He didn't hear my voice nor did he speak to me. As the appointment ended, he said that he didn't need to hear from me unless I wanted any of these tests or had new symptoms. I left the office, wanting to return to my old neurologist and to see my psychotherapist.

Three weeks later, I found myself making phone calls to New York City, trying to identify a new doctor for my father, who had Alzheimer's disease. In the middle of dialing the phone, I stopped myself. There was something wrong here. I could take care of my father, but not myself. I'd been here before.

It was time to call Mike Gardner, the local neurologist who friends and colleagues had recommended and who shared an office with Dr. Kelly. I scheduled an appointment, explaining that I had seen his colleague but didn't feel comfortable with him. And I let Patty, the receptionist, know that I wasn't someone who fired doctors as a rule. Why did I need to defend myself?

Dr. Gardner was a handsome, soft-spoken man. He first asked about me, not the illness. He looked at me intently and showed an interest in my work, counseling others with illness and disability. He wanted to know my family history, and perked up when I spoke of my father's Alzheimer's. On the exam, he saw a nystagmus — a jerking of the eye — and explained that my fatigue and eye pain were a result of my eyes' inability to track together. I easily asked him questions, because he saw a person, not an object. When I asked Dr. Gardner about the possible course of my MS and what explanations he could give for its recent moderation, he explained that as some women with MS approach menopause, their hormonal cycles alter and their MS symptoms stabilize.

We related person to person. The cartoon on his office wall of a patient kicking the neurologist out the window when he tested for reflexes indicated that this doctor understood, or at least tried to understand, the patient's experience. This is what I need to help me live with the uncertainty that is MS.

As we left his office, Dr. Gardner asked me to make an appointment in six months, but to call before then if I had any troubling symptoms. We agreed that an MRI might be warranted if and when my symptoms changed. The first neurologist had seen a body. This man saw a person.

Decision '97
April 2006

I didn't want to go there. But everyone told me to: the National MS Society, my current neurologist — "I think it's time to consider the options," he said gently — and even my former neurologist. The new interferon medications for MS, Betaseron and Avonex, had been approved by the FDA in 1993 and 1996. Over and over again, I heard that these drugs were the first to make a real difference in treating MS. They limited both the number of flare-ups ("exacerbations" in medical terminology) and their intensity.

Yet I was frustrated that no one could explain to my lay mind exactly how the interferons — proteins made by the body — work. MS is an autoimmune disease; my immune system unpredictably attacks the myelin sheath surrounding my nerves. Somehow, one of the interferons — interferon beta — would slow that down. Beyond that, I was lost. I worried that there were adverse reactions that the drug company had not yet uncovered, and that despite evidence to the contrary, Avonex would increase the risk of cancer or some such thing. I'd been anxious all my life. I knew how to look for the alligator in the closet, whether one was there or not.

I called my former neurologist in Boston, desperately trying to resolve my debate. "No one can predict your course of MS, but we do know that the new medications stop progression for most people."

I still didn't want to go there. But how could I not?

After no flare-ups for five years, I had been astonished by one the previous year — both eyes had lost their peripheral vision for a few weeks — and now this May, my arms and legs had become spastic. Despite all this, I wanted to deny that my MS could get worse. I'd had MS for more than fifteen years; the first five had been bad — frequent flare-ups led to loss of strength and coordination in my arms, hands, and legs and impaired my walking. My eyes, after several bouts of optic neuritis and double vision in the 1980s, now tired easily. But I'd been fairly stable for more than ten years. Flare-ups had been infrequent and I bounced back more quickly from them.

I asked myself, why mess with success? Why jab myself with a needle each week? Why risk the flu-like side-effects that the interferon medications caused? How much could my body take? My neurologist had warned me that exacerbations often increased in intensity over time. I wanted to be the exception to that rule. Was I fooling myself? My whole-body fatigue, which is the hallmark of MS, had been getting worse over the last couple of years. The flare-up in May had been frightening. One day, on my morning walk, my right leg wouldn't lift up from the ground. The right arm wouldn't keep my cane in place. Over the next few weeks, this weakness and spasticity intensified. But after a mild course of steroids, my body returned to itself, again convincing me — or was it deceiving me? — that my MS was special; it would take a different, more benign, course.

I had a good life. I lived in a neighborhood of people who knew and cared about each other. After seven years of marriage, my husband, Jim, and I were still deeply in love. My work as a psychotherapist was fulfilling. Now I feared that my ordered world would come crashing down if I tampered with it. I wanted to control things that I could not. I longed to be at peace with this decision, yet trust and faith eluded me.

I knew there were some deeper feelings that I was avoiding. So I called my psychotherapist, whom I hadn't seen for a few years. When I hung up the phone after making an appointment for the next day, I burst into tears. I had begun to glimpse those feelings. I didn't want to have MS, and felt angry that I had to make this decision, that my body needed a stupid drug. I wanted to believe that my MS would never hurt me again. It felt like I was getting diagnosed once more.

When I discovered this sadness, I began to let go of trying to control my MS. That summer, I read Tarot cards, talked with friends, and just sat with it all. I took my first dose of Avonex on September 12, 1997. I've had no new MS symptoms since that day nine years ago. Each week, I assist my husband by ripping the paper wrapping off the Band-Aid while Jim rubs alcohol on the injection site and gives me the shot. I still hate that injection; its painful jab is too real to minimize. Yet the flu-like symptoms have been mild; a headache might linger for some hours, but nothing more. I have more energy and my body is in much better shape than it was two decades ago when I was newly diagnosed. I don't know if it's the medication that has made the difference, but now I can live with that unknown.

LOSS AND CHANGE

To Knit or Not to Knit
Spring 2003

My older sister was expecting her first child in the summer of 1985; her due date was August 18. We knew it was a boy, and I wanted to knit him a baby blanket. In May, I bought skeins of soft aqua-colored yarn.

I hadn't knit anything for several years before sitting down with this project. My mother had taught me to knit when I was a child, but I was never very good. I knit my father a scarf when I was about ten. "It was very long and skinny and not of much use," my mother says, "or maybe it was a misshapen sweater." So much for my skill. But when I was a teenager, I did succeed at making colorful scarves that triumphed as gifts, or at least I thought they did. At age twenty-nine I figured I could make a simple baby blanket.

There was a catch, however. I had been diagnosed with multiple sclerosis in December 1981. MS is an unpredictable but nonfatal disease of the central nervous system. Functions such as seeing and walking become uncontrolled because messages to and from the brain don't get through correctly. Since my diagnosis, I had had several flare-ups of the illness. For a few weeks, I'd experience lack of coordination or balance, difficulty walking, or impaired vision, all with extreme fatigue. These episodes were scary; I could become unable to walk or lose my vision entirely — or neither of these things could happen.

I have the "relapsing-remitting" form of MS, but that phrase is misleading. During an exacerbation in May 1983, I had lost my coordination. I felt as if I were wearing boxing gloves and I couldn't tie my shoes or write my name. Now, two years later, even "in remission" I still had difficulty writing. The fluid pen strokes I made when rested became a jerky scrawl when I was tired. Ah, these were the "residual" symptoms that my neurologist had described.

Even as I accepted the reality of MS, I often felt fine. The support of my friends and family sustained me. My physician's optimism rubbed off on me. During my most desperate times, I heard her words, "This, too, will pass." She had no idea if my MS would progress rapidly, but statistics gave us hope. Two-thirds of people with MS are still walking twenty-five years after diagnosis.

Living with chronic illness is about making choices about how to respond to the problem. When weary, I can either trust my own judgment and rest, or ignore my gut and skip my nap. I was dealt a lousy hand of cards, but how I play them is under my control.

With a mix of anxiety and excitement, I chose to begin a program in social work in September 1984. I loved the work. The fatigue that is the hallmark of MS slowed me down and demanded that I pace myself, but I managed to keep up with my studies.

In July 1985 I had just completed my first year of school and was recovering from a mild episode of blurred vision. I had begun the baby blanket in June but had to put it aside because of the visual problems. Knitting did not come easily. It was not just that I had lost fine motor skills. Over the last few years, I had discovered that the simplest tasks could enervate me — cutting an apple, reading a newspaper, even watching television. The damage to my optic nerve from episodes of double vision meant that using my eyes for anything might exhaust me. My eyes could become heavy and tight, as if someone or something was pinching them. We don't realize how much our visual sense orients us to the world until we start to lose it.

I had begun to rest my eyes periodically by closing them in order to avoid visual stimulation. At school, when tired, I would lie down on a couch with my eyes shut between classes. Afterwards, my eyes would return to normal. I learned quickly that summer that knitting is not just about manual dexterity. We use our eyes, too.

My neurologist told me that people with MS use ten times the energy that other people do to conduct their nerves' messages. No wonder knitting exhausted me! I would knit two - purl two for ten minutes, and then need to lie down for five. But damn it, I was determined to finish this blanket for the first child of the next generation.

That summer's exacerbation interrupted me briefly, but when the symptoms remitted, I resumed work on the blanket. I wondered if my vision and fine motor skills would allow me to finish it.

At this point in my life, I didn't know if I would ever have children of my own. Between MS and graduate school, I had little time to pay attention to the dating scene. And children? If and when I met my mate, MS fatigue would cause me to think long and hard about that prospect. But I was excited by my sister's pregnancy. She had not hesitated about her decision. As I began to knit again for her baby, I wove the excitement of anticipation and a feeling of tenderness for mother and child into each stitch. I knit slowly but diligently.

We welcomed Benjamin into the world on August 27, 1985. I was still knitting.

That fall, classes resumed. Time and energy were at a premium. But perseverance and patience won out. On Thanksgiving Day, I presented the blanket to Ben and his parents. It was so much more than a blanket to me. It was a triumph of body and soul.

It is eighteen years later and I haven't picked up knitting needles since. But as I write this story, I've decided to try to knit again. I want to rediscover the skill and how it affects me. It's like riding a bicycle, I tell myself. Some things you just never forget. My hands know the motions well. Cast on, put needle in stitch, lift arm, bring yarn over and towards me, pull needle through. But my arms feel heavy; my eyes fatigue quickly. I recognize that I have made a choice. I will no longer knit, even though I am still able.

I have a good life as a psychotherapist, writer, and speaker, with a husband, good friends, and two cats. Benjamin is about to go away to college and I still have a skein of the aqua yarn. Sometimes I use the yarn as a cat toy, or I use it sparingly when needed to mend a sweater, darn a sock, or wrap a present.

But far more importantly, I save the yarn to remind me of what is possible.

Off Balance in Body and Mind
August 2003

I fell last week. It scared the hell out of me. I was coming down the hill from my house, taking a step down from the grass onto the pavement. I was late for a Friday evening potluck at the neighborhood's common house. The summer had been quiet around here — children off to camp, friends and families vacationing at the beach or in the mountains — and I looked forward to hanging out with my neighbors.

Momentum sped me quickly down the hill. I wore sandals that offered little support but were useful for short trips around the neighborhood, and I carried a pottery bowl, brimming with red cherries. I stepped down from the grass onto the pavement, a step that was too big for me. As I made that stride, I lost my balance. I started toppling to the left and let go of the bowl to free my hands. My feet were fifteen inches from the ground. I fell on my left side, my weak side. It's the left leg that is heavy and stiff and the left side of my face that tingles and feels like the skin is being stretched, all symptoms of my multiple sclerosis. It was probably the left leg that collapsed as I stepped down.

I didn't have time to think about any of this. I only had half a second to feel terror and pray that I would be okay. What I still can hear clearly is the bang of my head as it hit the pavement and my thought, "This is going to be bad." It's amazing how much can go through your mind in an instant. I lay on the pavement for a few seconds and waited for the bleeding to begin or to lose consciousness. But I didn't pass out. I felt my scalp for blood but felt none. I turned to look at my leg, but there was only broken, red skin.

I sat up, shaking, and heard my husband, running up the hill. Jim called out my name with alarm, "Dana! I heard a crash!" He came up to me and I responded in a shaky voice, "I'm okay." I put my arms around him, and tears of fear and relief followed. Several neighbors came out from the potluck. I looked up at their faces and again, in a shaky voice, said, "I'm okay." "Thank goodness," my neighbor Sue responded. Yes.

Neighbors began to pick up the cherries that were still rolling on the asphalt. Michel, an artist, commented on the beautiful bowl. He picked up the shards, looked at me and said, "I will create something with these for you." I was touched by his generosity and warmth. My neighbors circled around me. I saw fear in their faces, or maybe it was all still in me.

Silently, I began to blame myself for this near disaster. Stop carrying things around the neighborhood. You shouldn't wear these sandals anymore. And stop taking that shortcut; walk a safer way and avoid the big step. At least, don't do all these things at once.

I began to realize that I was hiding my fear by covering it with self-blame. Instead, I decided I could change some habits and thoughts. I turned to Sue, who still stood near me, and said that I would use my cane more often. "I don't often see you with your cane," she replied. I explained that I didn't usually need it for short walks, but used it when I walked into town and for my fast morning walks around the neighborhood. I began to wonder if I ever avoided using the cane because of what others might think. What would be your first impression? Would you judge or label me? How much was my own judgment? I had thought I no longer cared how others perceived me and my disability, but I had to admit there were times when I did.

Falling is my greatest fear with MS. I know that anyone can fall, but I'm more at risk with my poor balance and weak legs.

And years of steroid treatment for the MS have made my bones brittle.

Within the last week, I have stopped taking that shortcut with the big step and I limit what I carry in the neighborhood. I've put the sandals in the back of my bedroom closet. And I'm letting go of what others think, because those cares put me off balance.

Hanging on to Hope
December 2003

I walk into Dan and Sue's home. My left eye is throbbing. Eye pain, a recurring symptom of multiple sclerosis for me, has lingered for two days. I look to the right, into the kitchen. Brownies and a cake sit on the counter. My eyes sting and my eyelids are heavy. In my peripheral vision, sparks of light flash.

These are familiar sensations. When I'm recovering from an MS exacerbation or have just swum in tepid water, when I'm in a room full of noise and light or am fatigued in some way, my eyes react.

I'm scared. I don't know what will come next. Right now, there are fireworks all around me. I should go back home. But I don't. I am drawn towards people, away from the isolation I both crave and despise.

My neighbor Jude sees me and asks how I am. "Still recovering from Thanksgiving. It was wonderful, but it was too much for me," I say as I walk into the kitchen.

Thank goodness, there are only four people here so far. Dan has invited neighbors over to share his birthday cake. But it's the end of a holiday weekend and maybe others have also had enough.

"Sit down," Jude insists. "You know that hosting Thanksgiving can tire anyone."

"I've been doing nothing all weekend but lying on my couch and listening to WCRB," I respond.

"I wish I could do that," Jude offers. "The idea of listening to classical music escapes me, just when I need it most."

More people enter the room — Jane, Michel, Harriett, Bob. I sit at the kitchen counter, not wanting to move, lest I lose my seat. Jude's ten-year-old twin girls, Ali and Jenna, come upstairs from the basement. Their bubbly presence always brings a smile to my face. Even this evening.

All of a sudden, the kitchen seems crowded. I still haven't moved from my seat. Familiar faces float by me — Marcia and her son Kenyon and Dan and Sue's children, Alex and Rebecca. Sue lights the birthday cake. I look away from the flickering candles. Voices fill the air with the familiar song. A piercing child's voice — Alex is excited for his father — screams the "Happy Birthday" refrain in my ears. "Shhh...," Sue urges her son. Other adults are cringing, too. Sometimes it's not just me who gets overwhelmed.

I welcome the cake. Although I limit my intake of fat, this is a lemon cake, so I accept Sue's offer of it. I fantasize that foods I usually avoid will cure my eye pain.

The cake melts in my mouth. The lemon taste tingles on my tongue. The sugar comforts me. My eye still throbs.

"Let's go into the living room," Sue invites us. It's the children's cue to return to the basement. The adults find comfortable seats on the sofa and chairs. "I'll just lie on the floor with my eyes closed," I say, wondering if I should just go home. I want to be around people, but my heavy eyes make me self-conscious. Lying down feels so good, though. I forget what others might think.

Sue teaches us to play the game of "psychiatrist."

"One person is the psychiatrist and leaves the room," she begins. Marcia volunteers for that role and walks back into the kitchen. "Marcia has to figure out what illness we all have," Sue explains. Damn. I can't get away from it. I'm so self-involved that it takes me some moments to realize that Sue doesn't mean a physical illness. I let go of my self-conscious concerns and enjoy my prone position, surrounded by friends.

I stay for one round of the game and then realize that it's time for me to go home. I feel dizzy as I rise from the floor and head towards the front door. Again, I'm scared by my disorientation. I shuffle back to the living room and murmur to my husband that I may need help walking the short distance home. "I'm here if you do," Jim says. When I step outside into the cold air, I feel refreshed. I start to walk and regain my bearings. But I know it's time for bed.

Walking home, I ask myself why I went to this event that made me so aware of my discomfort and difference. And I know the answer: To hang on to the hope that life is more than my pain. To know that though I may feel different from those around me, I'm not so different.

Mirrors of Loneliness
February 2006

I struggled with loneliness this week. I was feeling dizzy and fatigued from MS. Scared, too. It had been a while since I had experienced this intensity of symptoms. I spent a day at home, part of it in bed and disconnected from my colleagues, my friends, myself. That evening I felt a little better, so to salve my lonely wounds, I went to a neighborhood meeting, looking for comfort. But I didn't tell anyone of my day's struggles. In the middle of the gathering, when I longed to be lying down at home with a good book, I realized what I had done. To stave off loneliness, I had forced myself to be with people, but that was the loneliest place to be. My silence cut me off from my friends and myself. At home alone, I could have enjoyed solitude, a confident and centered place. But I had been scared to be with myself.

The next day, I felt fine. My energy was back. My eye fatigue was all but gone. Once more, I felt connected with friends. But I wondered what role my lack of self-acceptance had played in my loneliness. Had I created a wall around me through which no one could penetrate? I couldn't help but wonder if my silence about my symptoms had reinforced my loneliness. And if my fear at being alone was a rejection of the me with MS.

I emailed some friends, soliciting thoughts about their experience of loneliness and solitude. Not surprisingly, most people wanted to talk in person. Perhaps it was painfully ironic to write emails about loneliness. The impersonal nature of email isolates its writer. This topic needed the human voice. So we talked.

Carol was recovering from cardiac surgery and coping with its accompanying exhaustion. "Loneliness is the absence of necessary empathy," she said. "From others or from yourself?" I asked. Carol admitted that she did judge herself harshly for her slow recovery. But I know from my clients and myself that ill people and healthy people withdraw from one another. We all feel too scared or too helpless. It leaves us lonely, because our culture doesn't teach any of us to embrace ourselves or others who are ill.

Becky reflected on her loneliness fifty years ago as an adolescent. "The most profound lonely experience for me was being gay as a teenager. I felt so helpless. I wanted so badly to be straight." She still remembered the Baptist church in her town, which made it clear that homosexuality was a sin. Part of her loneliness was feeling isolated and different from her friends. "There was nowhere I could communicate safely, and I longed to be heard," she continued. But her loneliness remained when, as an adult, she walked into another church where she could have been heard. This one was in Cambridge and full of hundreds of lesbians. "It contradicted my way of being in the world. It was so hopeful, yet so frightening. What if this thing I had been yearning for was not really what I wanted after all? And if all these lesbians were around, how come I'd never met them? Feeling lonely in this crowd was more lonely than being alone."

Yvonne contrasted her sense of self in loneliness and in solitude. "In loneliness, I'm reaching out for something or someone, but the connection is absent within myself and with the other." Her loneliness was both an unfulfilled yearning and a disconnection from herself. "But my solitude is a mirror," Yvonne continued. "It lets me see what I need and feel and that I can extend myself without losing myself."

"I love being alone," said Becky. "In solitude, I nourish myself. I feel confident there." Similarly, another friend remarked that in being alone and lonely when she lived abroad, she learned to value her separateness. "Feeling good about myself and feeling known counteracted my loneliness. And when I felt a strong connection to myself, I enjoyed my solitude."

In loneliness, we can feel sad or we can feel angry. Sad at the loss of our role in the world or at the rejection because we are different — gay or ill or the new kid on the block. Angry that our body has failed us or that others are not there for us. And the sadness and anger disguise each other. "I can get angry when I feel lonely, because I want to hide my sadness," said Becky. "I don't want to show my vulnerability. I'll get hurt." Is the anger a way to stay connected with others, or does the resentment at unmet needs leave us alone again with ourselves?

Loneliness is an unfulfilled longing for connection. We can fulfill that longing by first accepting our state and connecting with ourselves, and then find a way to genuinely connect with others. Sometimes the world is not a friendly place for people who are different. Sometimes, we try to hide our differences and end up feeling isolated. Always, the way through is to face the challenge of accepting where we are and who we are.

Stories of Madness
September 2005

The First Story:
Growing up in our families, maybe we were hurt by anger, or maybe anger was unspoken, or both. Now, we all stumble and land as best we can. My father had a temper. His three children have inherited some of it.

I was stuck in traffic, traveling to Northampton with my husband for a psychotherapists' workshop at Smith College when my anger visited. We were more than an hour away from our destination, and the workshop began in half an hour. And now, during the morning rush hour, I saw miles of cars ahead of me.

"Uh-oh, Jim. This could be bad," I said. I became silent, but I was slowly fuming inside, as traffic on Route 290 refused to move. Knowing that Jim hated it when I yelled, I said in a tight voice, "Jim, I want to yell and blame you for all this." Never mind that he had reviewed the route with me and we had agreed on it. I had to blame something to control the mess we were in.

Jim responded, "Okay, thanks for the warning. Try the yelling for ten minutes."

So I began. "Damn, I hate this!" I screamed, as you can in a car. "Stop! This is so unfair. I want to blame you, but I can't! I want us to turn around, but we can't. We're trapped! Why is this happening?" I pounded the dashboard, glimpsed the physical violence that could accompany anger — the rage — and got scared. I grew silent, seething inside.

I tried to say a serenity prayer to myself, but I was too angry to even remember the words. It's just a workshop, for goodness' sake, I thought. For mental health professionals, no less. You should do better than this. Should I? I looked at the clock. No way would we get there on time. Another "Damn," and more, came out of me.

We'd traveled for an hour, but we'd gone only ten miles. I burst out, "I hate that I needed you to drive me!" The anger melted into sadness. "If I didn't have to care about my energy, I would have driven myself yesterday and come home whenever," I said. My rage turned to tears as I spoke about the ways that MS limits me. Hiding behind that wall of anger was sadness. I'd found it.

The Second Story:
You are angry at your spouse. He has forgotten to do the dishes. Or she has left the bedroom in a mess. Or he has worked late too many nights in a row. You feel misunderstood and abandoned. But you remain silent, ashamed of your sensitivity, scared of where your anger might take you. The shame leads you to hide these parts of yourself. Your anger builds. It's a vicious cycle with anger: you're ashamed or afraid of the feelings — they are so uncomfortable — that you hide them from others. The silence reinforces the shame, causing the anger to simmer and grow. The anger intensifies and the cycle begins again. But one day, you can no longer tolerate the tension.

"I'm doing it again," you say to your spouse. "I'm stuffing my anger, unwilling to acknowledge it with you. It's driving us apart." After a few moments, your partner replies, "You finally said something. I was feeling angry and powerless. I didn't know what to do, so I just ignored you." Naming the anger and the problem lessens the intensity of the emotion, and somehow allows the two of you to connect.

We've all traveled somewhere on this continuum of anger — with the fear or the shame. Or maybe we've felt powerless over a situation and anger became our outlet. Or maybe we couldn't tolerate our fear or sadness, so we moved to anger.

The Third Story:
My friend Sally told me about the anger she has felt with her daughter, Debbie. "I yell. Loudly," said Sally. "I say things that I wish I hadn't said. Then I have to clean it up."

"It's a momentary burst of power, a self-justification," she continued. "It's an attempt to control the other. And it's a judgment of the other. I'm right, you're wrong. I feel out of control. I talk with Debbie after my outbursts about the 'mean mommy' who visited. It's not me."

We're angry the most at those we love the most. The anger is hidden, then revealed. Either no one gets hurt, or we do what we can to make it right. Then we stumble on to fear, relief, sadness, or whatever is next.

CULTURE AND STIGMA

The She That Is Me
June 2003

It is July 1983. I live in Waltham, Massachusetts, and teach history at a private high school.

One night, I wake up and start walking towards the bathroom. I feel intense tingling sensations in my feet as I totter out of the bedroom. I worry that this is another exacerbation of multiple sclerosis, the illness that has startled me for the last two years. Or am I just groggy and out-of-it because it's three a.m.?

I wobble back to bed but have trouble falling back to sleep. What is going on inside me? I obsess about my body — I want to control it — but finally cry myself to sleep.

The next morning, my fears are confirmed. When I try to get out of bed, I can't feel my feet on the floor at all. I don't know where my body is in space. Close to nine o'clock, I call my neurologist and make an appointment. She will see me that afternoon and confirm that this is MS. I have lost my balance. I have lost my innocence.

That night, I cry myself to sleep again. I am terrified. Friends have brought me dinner and helped me to laugh, but still, when they leave, I am alone, in a body estranged.

The next day, I start to compensate. I hold on to furniture in my apartment, the first floor of a two-story house. I call the local chapter of the MS Society. Three hours later, Debra, the support services director, comes over to loan me a walker. It will help me balance and get around, if I'm willing to use it.

Debra's visit and generosity warm me. As she leaves, I finally notice that outside my door, the sky is a cloudless blue. I want to get out of my house and not let my body imprison me. I step onto the porch and gingerly go down the stairs, grabbing the porch railing with one hand and dragging my walker with the other as it bumps down the seven steps. When I had looked for an apartment the previous year, it hadn't occurred to me that I wouldn't be able to navigate stairs.

I stand in my driveway and face the road with my walker in front of me. I discover that I am trembling. It is my self-image, not trust in my physical ability, that is shaken. I fear what others will think of me. What do I look like, holding on to this walker for balance? It disgusts me. Twenty-seven years old, I'm supposed to be in fine health. Aren't people who use walkers either elderly or mentally retarded? I am dismayed to recognize my assumptions and prejudices. Young teens walk by my driveway and gaze at me — or is it through me? Do they see me or the freak I believe I am? They laugh as they easily walk on. Don't mistake me for a retard, I want to shout. Then I gulp with shame for such thoughts. An older couple walk by and also stare, but then they nod and smile, acknowledging my presence. Later, it occurs to me that they might understand, because they also know human frailty. They are not as afraid as I imagine the teenagers are, or as I am.

Slowly, I walk down my driveway to the road. Lift the walker and my foot, move them forward, place them down and step. Balance! If I ever get it back, I will cherish it.

I reach the sidewalk and take a left, aiming to go around the block. Slowly, I pass the Catholic church. Its stoic silence encourages me to pause. Then I continue to lift and step. I am getting the hang of this walking.

I see my reflection in a store window and stop suddenly. I am outside myself, looking in. Seeing myself so starkly, needing the walker, I feel pity. I don't want to see this vulnerability.

I am back at my driveway, exhausted. I lift and step on the drive. When I get to the porch stairs, I look around but see no one. I sit down and push myself up the stairs, again dragging the walker with me. I stand, lift, and step through the door into the living room, and collapse on the couch.

That day, I begin a course of Prednisone. This is my third MS exacerbation in five months. In March, my legs felt heavy and stiff; I walked like a robot — gingerly, yet mechanically. In May, I lost my coordination; with my hands feeling huge and clumsy, I couldn't tie my shoes or hold a pen. Those symptoms have remitted almost entirely, but I am overwhelmed by this constant onslaught. My loss of balance has uprooted my identity, the person who I believe I am.

I call my brother in New York. I cry and ask him what I did to bring on this exacerbation. I have turned my fear and anger at this illness against myself and into self-blame. Adam reminds me that the illness is not my fault; this flare-up is probably due to the position of the constellations in the sky. Skeptic that he is, his humor helps me to test my reality and to reconnect with some vital part of me. I am reminded that relationships sustain me.

The next week, my balance begins to return in more ways than one. I can move around my apartment with greater ease, although I still use the walker when I venture outdoors. Now, I smile at others on the street. I notice the trees and the birds, more than what strangers may perceive.

Towards the end of July, I visit Adam and his wife in upstate New York. The rest and relaxation and the support of loved ones soothe my body and soul. I start to let go of judgments of myself and my body. I talk and cry about my losses and fears. I begin to admire the cane that a carpenter-friend has made me. Over and over again, I'm learning what I can control and what I can't.

I've begun to grieve. Running away from my grief that summer day with the walker estranged me from myself. I was fighting the MS, not learning new ways to respond to the illness. In my attempt to deny my own negative self-judgments, I imagined that others had those biases. I have to let go of my own and society's prejudice in order to accept myself.

The next year, I decide to attend social work school. I want to help others deal with the loss and vulnerability that encompasses life. My studies and psychotherapy help me to understand myself. I read *Stigma* by Erving Goffman, the renowned sociologist, and see the interplay between my own self-image and society's projections. I continue to grow up.

Twenty years later, I tell the story of how my prejudices dared to challenge my self-image. I skirted dangerously close to self-loathing on that summer day. When I walk past a store window now with my cane, the woman smiling back understands. I am no longer outside myself — she is me.

The Hierarchy of Disability
December 1999

The other morning, a reporter called me to apologize for a possible error of information in the newspaper. She thought she might have written that I had muscular dystrophy, instead of multiple sclerosis. My reactions surprised me. I thought, if I must have a disability, let me keep this one. MS is more romantic, more feminine than muscular dystrophy. Barbara Jordan and Joan Didion are my role models. Not that I want a chronic illness, but after almost twenty years, I'm used to MS.

I thought, what will people think of me if they believe I have muscular dystrophy? Isn't it worse than MS, more life-threatening? The need for a wheelchair more certain? They would think, "How unusual, it's rare for a woman to have MD." As a psychotherapist, I try to help clients to separate themselves from the thoughts and feelings about illness that dominate our culture, to accept their needs and develop a solid self-image, to reject the notion that "I am my illness."

Yet here I was, worrying about what people might think. I projected my prejudice and unfounded horror of an illness onto others, imagining that my thoughts would be theirs. The recognition of my actions gave me empathy for my clients who struggle with the attitudes of friends and family. I could also now understand the able-bodied who anger me, because I, too, had perceived people with an illness as pariahs, outcasts. Ironically, I labeled and feared those with MD, trying to put myself above them, as if there was a hierarchy of disability. Even I was trying to maintain emotional distance from illness, running away from my fear and vulnerability.

The irony is that some might fear multiple sclerosis more than they do other illnesses. Yet I've learned to manage my life with MS. My professional life grows from my personal experience. MS is an emotional challenge as much as a physical one. Fatigue limits my activities. I've lost coordination in my hands, strength and balance in my legs. Double vision pays a visit at times. The unpredictability of these symptoms is scary; I could become blind or paralyzed, temporarily or permanently. Or none of these things might ever happen.

What did I mean by thinking that one illness is "worse" than another? That it makes one less happy? Receive a kind of pity that is unwanted? Does the fear of life in a wheelchair stem from the dread of dependency in our culture? Does the burden of illness and disability make our lives less valuable? Or do we offer others the opportunity to learn about intimacy and vulnerability without running away?

There was no error in the newspaper. The article stated that I did, indeed, have multiple sclerosis. But I learned some things. Even those of us with disability compare ourselves to one another. "At least, I'm able to walk" can give me a false sense of superiority. Someone else might look at my life and say, "At least, I have the energy for child-rearing."

The hope is that we can witness and honor the experience of others, whatever that may be. After the diagnosis those twenty years ago, I immediately went to the home of a good friend to tell him I had multiple sclerosis. He responded, "Oh, now you'll be one of Jerry's kids!" His attempt at humor relaxed us, but I remember thinking, "No, that's muscular dystrophy. My experience is going to be of MS and let's understand that."

So the other day, prejudice reared its ugly head. I saw first-hand how fear and ignorance can develop into negative attitudes. And I'm supposed to be above all that, considering my personal and professional experience. Ha! I understand more fully now how confronting biases can go a long way towards overcoming prejudice.

Not Always So Black and White
January 2001

The story of Casey Martin, a golfer with a disability, has captured my attention. Because I so understand his predicament. A federal appeals court ruled last year that Martin was entitled to use a golf cart rather than walk the course on the PGA Tour. His right leg is so atrophied and weak from a circulatory disorder, Klippel-Trenaunay-Weber syndrome, that walking the length of a golf course is impossible. The PGA Tour, which has a no-cart rule for its circuit, responded by taking its case to the Supreme Court.

Some commentators have said that the sports world should be exempt from protections for people with disabilities. Despite the increased visibility of women's sports, the athletic arena does have a tradition of being a macho world; inclusion is not its top priority. If you combine this with the fact that golf is a sport that cherishes rules and tradition, then Martin loses out. But the fact is that, disabled or not, Martin is a star. He has a strength that calls for recognition. He is not a very good walker, but he is a great golfer.

It is possible that you doubt Martin. It may be hard to understand how he can swing a golf club with expertise yet be unable to walk to the next tee. You might also wonder how Martin can stand and flex his knees without problem but find walking so difficult that he must ask for this exception. His talents might make you question the severity of his condition. Illness and disability might scare you so (because none of us is immune) that you just don't want to believe Martin. If he had a significant disability, could he really compete in sports with the able-bodied?

But disability is not always so black and white. We had a president who used a wheelchair, even if he and the world tried to hide that fact. Sometimes disability is invisible. People who "look so well" with lupus or multiple sclerosis may function quite well at work or home, but they can't help but be affected by the fatigue in their bodies. Even with MS for the last twenty years, I can climb mountains with my cane, but I use a wheelchair in museums to avoid the pain and exhaustion that come from standing. I understand how Casey Martin can move his body perfectly to play golf but not to walk.

What often harms people with disabilities is not their "handicap," but the world's attitudes. If Casey Martin is such a great golfer, why not let him use a cart? Let's use the Americans with Disabilities Act (ADA) to level the playing field.

Martin's case reminds me of the debate in the Appalachian Mountain Club about whether to make their White Mountain huts in New Hampshire accessible. Some think it ridiculous to build ramps and have accessible bathrooms on mountains that are five thousand feet high. I did at first. But there are hikers in wheelchairs who, with assistance and a lot of determination, have made it to the top in glory. Haven't they earned access to a warm bed and a tasty meal?

Martin was dealt a lousy hand (or leg) of cards, but he plays it well. We may want to peg him into the stereotype of "the hero who can overcome anything." But Martin, a former golf champion at Stanford University, only wants to continue to compete in the sport that he has played all his life. Requiring him to be a hero is hurtful to him and the thousands with disabilities who live life as best they can. It is unjust to demand a standard from them of constant courage and heroism.

These cases confuse me, however. Right and wrong are not clear-cut. Do we use limited financial resources to make places accessible in remote locations? If only one person in a wheelchair gets to the mountaintop, does that warrant an accessible entrance? Is it fair to use the ADA to alter the terms of a sporting competition? Is the twenty-five miles that golfers have to walk fundamental to the game? If it is, then why do golf carts exist? Perhaps to make the game more equitable for all. Here is the irony.

People want sports to be a simple story without the complexities and ambiguities of everyday life. They want golf to be about Tiger Woods, not Casey Martin. But Woods and Martin played together at Stanford University. Why can't they play together in the PGA?

Illness, Lies, and the Television Version
May 2001

I share a chronic illness with the President of the United States. President Bartlet, of TV's "The West Wing," has multiple sclerosis. In remission for the last eight years, he has kept silent about his illness.

When I first watched this story unfold, I was stunned. That MS, an illness about which many are misinformed, could be portrayed with accuracy to the television public was remarkable. MS is often depicted as an illness that "strikes victims" who "end up in wheelchairs." That the illness varies widely from person to person — there are progressive, moderate, and benign courses — is often overlooked. Nor do the ambiguities of MS for those who "look so well" but feel so lousy get attention. It may have been unrealistic that someone who works long hours and has the most stressful job in the world could have an illness whose primary symptom is an exhausting fatigue. But it was exciting that millions of viewers could receive a fine education about illness, and life, from this drama.

I began to watch "The West Wing" with regularity. MS did not often figure in the weekly plots. The illness was important, but it was not a big deal. I became engaged with the characters on the President's staff. I was proud of C.J., his press secretary. A confident and personable woman, she was a role model for all female viewers. I was enamored with Charlie, the President's personal aide. He was the epitome of cool, not batting an eye at the President's idiosyncratic demands for the perfect Thanksgiving carving knife. When the character of Joey Lucas, played by Marlee Matlin, was introduced, I was tickled. A presidential pollster, Lucas happened to have a serious hearing impairment, as does Matlin. Again, we were given the message that disability does not have to dominate one's life.

In the last few weeks of the second season, the President's staff found out about the MS. Some felt betrayed; a few showed concern for Bartlet's health. All were anxious about the public's reaction. In the season's final episode, the President disclosed his condition to the world.

Did the President lie to the public through a sin of omission? How much of this politician's life did the public have the right to know? Did he have the right to keep private about an illness that can be degenerative in some, but that in him has been quiet and only a nuisance? It's a big deal to have a serious illness, but is it a big deal if you can still live a full and productive life? Sixty years after F.D.R., we still debate whether or not to acknowledge Roosevelt's wheelchair.

Truth and honesty are central subjects in American politics. The interpersonal complexities of hiding the truth parallel the political ramifications of keeping secrets. People with chronic illness often face the issue of disclosure. Some, living with invisible symptoms, choose to hide illness from friends and colleagues. They fear the loss of their companions or their jobs. But in shutting down this part of themselves, they lose the intimacy that genuine connection brings, and they deny a part of themselves. In this fictional drama, the President's pollster assessed the public's reaction before the disclosure. People overwhelmingly responded by rejecting a politician who developed a serious illness, demanding that he step down. Would this, in truth, be the case if the fictional scenario actually happened? Is it an irrational fear of the unpredictability of some illnesses that is at play, or is it a rational response to the restrictions that illness imposes? Can the lessons in compassion and living with limitations override the possibility that the illness might progress?

What I appreciate about how the MS has been handled in "The West Wing" is that it has not been the central issue of the show, even though it has been a serious matter. It is just part of life. Politically, the MS has highlighted issues of honesty and privacy. Spiritually, the show has confronted issues of loss and vulnerability. The second season's final episode also showed the President in mourning for his beloved secretary, who was killed by a drunk driver. The story went beyond the fears that can be raised by a single focus on the random nature of ill health. The President railed against God about the unfairness of haphazard events in the world. And doesn't such randomness confront us all?

To Tell or Not to Tell
March 2004

Last month, a colleague asked me to speak to a breast cancer support group about disclosing illness. Who do you tell — family, friends, colleagues? What do you tell — the details or the bare minimum? When do you tell — now or later, if the illness becomes more visible?

And how does it feel to tell? Do you feel guilty, that you have somehow done something wrong to deserve this, or do you feel ashamed, that you are tainted in some way? Does that shame affect who, how, and when you tell? Or do you feel angry at our culture, which makes it difficult for you to accept the illness, for shunning you in order to allow the able-bodied to keep their eyes closed? Or do you feel relief because the secret is out? Clearly, the issue of disclosure has many layers.

I still give thanks to my first neurologist, who helped me skip over any shame. She made it clear that I had done nothing wrong to bring on multiple sclerosis, that it was likely caused by a virus that had lain dormant in my body for years. The stress of teaching may have been the trigger, but no one really knew.

I told everyone that first year, 1981, including family, friends, and colleagues. It wasn't my style to hide from others and I wanted — no, needed — the support. Back then, you could be fired just because you were ill or disabled. It was just as well that I was naive; it allowed me to be myself. Holly, another teacher, gave me a hug when I told. I described the illness and explained that it was unpredictable, but not fatal. Telling others about the MS helped to make it real.

Of course, not everyone was warm and fuzzy. When I first realized that I couldn't control people's reaction to the MS, I felt powerless and angry. I remember telling one friend that my interest in social work school stemmed from a desire to help others who faced difficult life events. She was concerned that this meant that I was focused on the MS to the detriment of the rest of my life. I was hurt by what felt like an unsupportive response. It was a few weeks before I began to wonder if her fear and discomfort with illness had affected her reaction.

When I began to use a cane a few years later, I started to hide. I had learned that serious illness frightened people and that first impressions mattered. So sometimes I would wait to tell people about the MS, even hiding the cane on a first visit.

I was particularly uncertain about the issue of disclosure when I entered the dating scene. Since being diagnosed at age twenty-five, I had not dated. My close friends accepted my MS, but I was not ready for the exposure that dating would entail. I feared rejection, imagining that men would only see the MS, because that was all I saw. As I slowly integrated MS into my identity, I recognized that I was so much more than the illness. I realized that a guy's response said more about him than about me. Did his discomfort reflect an unease with difference and vulnerability? If he couldn't embrace the entire Dana, was he the man for me?

In 1987, a man I was dating asked me, "Do you want to go for a bicycle ride?" We had been on only one date, but we had talked easily. It wasn't love at first sight, but that was a good sign. Falling in love quickly often meant that I was falling in love with a fantasy, not a real person.

Now, he had called me for another date. "I don't ride bicycles much," I replied. "How about a walk in the woods?" he tried again. I gulped and said, "Sure, that sounds nice," and we arranged to walk around a local reservoir. I hung up and realized that this guy might find out about MS sooner than I had planned. I loved the outdoors and walking, but MS reduced my stamina. I did what I could, which some days was more than expected; other days, my legs demanded rest.

As we began our walk, I took my cane, collapsed like a tent pole and secured with a rubber band, out of my purse. I released the rubber band and the cane dramatically fell into place. "Meet my cane," I declared. "Oh, what's that for?" my date asked matter-of-factly. "I sometimes have trouble walking," I replied. "I have multiple sclerosis." I told him about MS, that symptoms could come and go for years, that my doctor was optimistic. We had walked about three-quarters of the way around the reservoir and sat down on a bench. "How are you doing with all this?" I asked. "It brings me down to earth. And you?" he asked. I talked about my nervousness, how I didn't mean to tell him so soon, but this was just my life.

Disclosure is a personal decision and a different one each time. It was scary to tell that day, but I'm glad I did. Seventeen years later, my husband and I still walk around ponds and ask each other, "How are you doing?"

Soft Tissues for the Rough Times
March 2005

Walking home one evening from a neighbor's house, I was oblivious to the frigid winter air, though the need to blow my nose was obvious. I got home and, sneezing, I scurried to find a box of tissues. This couldn't be the beginning of a cold, because mine always began with a sore throat and there was none of that tonight. Sure, my husband had a cold the week before, but I wasn't going to get sick. I was above all that.

The next morning was Saturday. I awoke with a stuffy nose and a headache. I told myself to take it easy. MS, an autoimmune disease, can get triggered when the body is fighting an infection. I didn't want my immune system to attack my nerve linings instead of the cold germs.

I was sluggish all weekend. I read a good mystery and avoided walking outdoors. My headache eased, but my need for tissues did not. I still didn't have a sore throat, not even a cough, so I started to think that the congestion would abate quickly. On Monday, I stayed home and wrote. As the week progressed, I left the house to see psychotherapy clients, and the headache returned. At night, my sleep was interrupted — the worst side-effect of all — by nose blowing, sneezes, and restlessness.

My MS symptoms of eye pain, spasticity, and fatigue intensified by the end of the week. I got scared. I realized I wasn't doing anybody any good by working and by denying my need to take care of myself. I'm usually good at taking it easy when I'm tired. But this time, I wanted to be strong and invulnerable to the world of illness. Weren't these the distorted thoughts and beliefs that I helped my clients to question? I thought that by now I had learned to ignore our culture's message that getting sick was one's fault. Yes, we have a responsibility to take care of ourselves as best we can. But no, part of me had fallen into the belief that if I were tough, I could ward off this cold. That vigor and health equaled strength. So was it weak to be sick?

It was this type of thinking combined with my diminished energy that took away my resilience. First, a reader criticized my writing. Then, I couldn't seem to help a client's depression. Who was I to think I had so much power, anyway? I did a good job of finding my failures and stewing in them.

The cold lingered into the following weekend and the headache returned, all exacerbating my MS symptoms. I stayed prone and did little on Saturday, and then started to feel human again on Sunday. My head cleared. I felt as I did when coming out of an MS flare-up. The world was a beautiful place. I was good to myself. I bought only "ultra soft" tissues for my sensitive, now-chapped nose. I scheduled a massage for Monday afternoon.

I wrote my friend and colleague Tracy, who also has MS, about the self-criticism. She could relate. "There's something so insidious and invisible about how a little bit more of illness or strain depletes what we are able to handle," Tracy wrote back. "And then we blame ourselves, when actually there's a very good reason, that has nothing to do with us, for feeling so horrible. When my body ails, it's not really ME that's failing: it's my body. And that I can forgive."

I thought about how we blame ourselves for illness, whether it is MS or a cold, in an attempt to control its origin and outcome. I have come to believe that there are aspects of illness that we cannot control, that have a life of their own. Some days, even when I feel rested, my legs still feel "gimpy," a word I use to describe my clumsiness and loss of coordination and balance.

But I can control how I respond to the illness and to my self-perceptions.

We learn about the meanings of health and illness at an early age. Recently, I had a conversation with an eleven-year-old neighbor who struggles with migraines. Jenna told me, "Every day when I wake up feeling well, I'm so happy. I congratulate myself for doing something right." I understood Jenna's glee. I've been there. But if we compliment ourselves for feeling well, how do Jenna and I avoid berating ourselves for feeling sick? By forgiving our bodies and ourselves, by learning what we can control and what we can't. And by storing away a few extra boxes of those ultra-soft tissues for the next cold.

Take Back Your Time
November 2005

Did you know that the United States military has a Directorate of Time? And a director of the Directorate of Time? Fantasize for a moment about what you might do in this position. I would stop all clocks for a day. Without warning. Instruct everyone to take one day off to chill. Most important, I would add an extra hour, every afternoon, for everyone to take a nap. And it would be my department's job to make sure that we all don't just return to our crazy, hectic lives. That would be my greatest challenge.

I've been struggling with time lately, because I've had the luxury of feeling well. So I do more — more work projects, more community tasks. Then I forget appointments, lose files. Trip on my way to the bathroom. With my extra energy, someone asks me if I've considered more play. I ponder that.

This week I study time and I know I'm not alone. James Gleick, in *Faster: The Acceleration of Just about Everything*, asserts that "We are in a rush. We are making haste." He writes that "the blacks," those punctuations between television shows "when the screen fades momentarily to darkness," are disappearing. We've lost our down time. Gleick proposes that "our ability to work fast and play fast gives us power," and that "behind all our haste lurks the fear of mortality." I ask myself: Is it the baby-boomers who are rushing things for fear we will lose our influence and run out of time?

I wonder how our speedy culture affects us. We no longer wait for postal mail, which we rename snail mail. Tasks multiply as we email, speed dial, fax, instant message. Fast forward, channel-surf. Ten seconds seems like an eternity. Does

our impatience affect our health? Do we still make time for
human connection? Have we become trapped in this electronic,
overloaded world? Do we have more leisure time or more time
to keep busy?

I connect with friends about their relationship to time. And
I find solutions. I'm struck that it is those with whom I speak,
not email, who help me the most. Yvonne, who says she's
always "wrestled with time more than anything else in my life,"
finds it helpful that our culture is so fast now. She's more
conscious of the pressure to speed up and more mindful to pace
herself. Living in community, she uses a neighbor to help her
account for time. They call each other in the morning, prioritize
their tasks for the next few hours, and then check back with
each other later in the day. "When I state my accomplishments,
I own what I've done and feel less overwhelmed," says Yvonne.
"I've taken back control and it slows me down."

Community helps me to pace myself, too. I run into my
neighbor Beth one Saturday, and we spontaneously connect and
take a walk. I leave my "to dos" behind at home and slow down
over supper with friends in our neighborhood's common house.

Carol, who is recovering from open heart surgery, speaks
with me about her lack of speed, a most difficult aspect of
healing. "I have to adjust to how slow I am. I never had to pace
myself before and I'm used to doing things quickly." She adds
in an email, "I don't think I'm judging myself critically, nor do
I think I'm wasting time. I'm definitely into accepting what
is…. I'm trying not to use energy to change what I can't."

Living with a chronic illness in this fast, busy culture, it's
taken me some time to accept that I must rest between tasks, lest
I receive a visit from overwhelming fatigue. Like Yvonne and
Carol, I realize that I can choose to reject our culture's pressure.

People with illness tell me that responding to the cultural
call for speed is one of their greatest challenges. "The faster I do

a task, the longer I have to lie down afterwards," says Jean, who has chronic fatigue syndrome. Frank, who has Parkinson's disease, says, "It takes so long for me to do things now. For a long time, I didn't want anyone to see that." Eating, dressing, or talking on the telephone are no longer simple tasks for these two. But Frank says that now, after five years, he appreciates his accomplishments like he never did. He also values the simple things — friends, family, relative health. Slowing down has allowed him to stop and smell the flowers.

If the director of the Directorate of Time doesn't give me that day off, I'll just take it anyway. It's about time.

LETTING GO

Just Like Life, Only More So
July 2004

It is clearly time for me to hone my basketball skills. There's a new basketball court in the neighborhood. One evening, I see ten-year-old Ali and Jenna and seven-year-old Tim shooting baskets. I can't resist asking if I can join in.

"Sure," they respond, though I hear notes of hesitation in their voices. I understand. This might be a joke.

In fact, I can't get the ball near the backboard. The kids are very solicitous. "Good job, Dana." "Really close." "Excellent," they call out to me. Didn't I say these words to them several years ago when they were just learning the game? How did the roles get reversed so quickly? I decide to leave the court to the kids for now, but vow to come back again soon when I can practice by myself.

A few days later, in a T-shirt and shorts, I stand on the small court. It is late afternoon and there's a threat of thunderstorms in the humid air. I grab one of the balls from a wooden crate and stand to the right of the basket. I dribble towards the hoop, bend my knees, and shoot. Again, the ball does not come close to the backboard. You used to be able to do this, I say to myself, remembering the days when I coached girls' basketball. Patience. My next shots are still way off. A few come closer; one even grazes the net, but I understand now that this will take some time.

Bill, a neighbor who does landscaping work, comes by to say hello. We chat. I say that I will shoot hoops until I make two baskets in a row, however long that takes; Bill intends to work outdoors, but the rumble of distant thunder has made him pause. I am confident that the rain will hold off. Bill asks about our neighbor who is ill. I am intent on shooting baskets and my response is minimal. I hope I don't seem rude, but basketball is my task right now. Bill doesn't seem to mind, for he goes on talking, asking my advice about how to communicate with this neighbor, while I continue to miss the hoop by a wide margin. Then he comments that basketball is all about angles. "It's really quite mathematical," he explains. "Get closer to the backboard and it will be easier." I try again and miss.

I feel frustrated. "You know I have MS, don't you?" "Yes," he replies. I wonder why I have any need to explain my poor play. Bill is so mild-mannered that I have no need to feel self-conscious.

"Do you want to take a shot?" I ask, bouncing him the ball. Casually, with one hand, mind you, he dribbles to the right of and close to the net and lobs one off the backboard. "Wow," I respond. I attempt his technique and the ball glides into the net. "Yahoo!" I exclaim. "Thanks, Bill."

Bill asks me if MS makes me hard on myself or controlling of others. The question challenges me, but I welcome it. I don't want MS to be a taboo subject.

I say, "I've learned to be good to myself and take it easy when I become fatigued. But sure, I can get controlling. When I can't climb on the stepstool to do a simple chore and have to wait for my husband to do it, that's frustrating. I'm angry that I can't do a simple task, so I want Jim to have done it yesterday. But you know, this isn't about illness. I was impatient and judged myself long before MS."

The conversation has distracted me momentarily from basketball. I return to the task at hand and remember Bill's advice to get close to the basket and use the angle. I want to succeed with those two shots in a row. The first one drops into the hoop. The next one doesn't. I begin to swear and then stop and remember to go easy on myself.

I say good-bye to Bill, who has decided to work outside after all, since the sun is shining brightly now. I shoot once more and miss.

Walking home, I ponder the ways in which illness has forced me to confront my demons — the impatient and controlling ones — and I remember that we all have our rough spots. Handling them is a matter of angles, and patience. MS is just like life, only more so.

A Challenge to Let Go
June 2002

I am unsure what I believe in. Maybe that makes me an agnostic. I do believe in letting go, that to believe we control all events and outcomes is a recipe for disaster. When I was diagnosed with MS in my mid-twenties, I watched my body shut down with its loss of coordination and vision. I perseverated on my body's collapse, thinking that if I focused constantly on these changes, I could, magically, will them away. Eventually they did go away for a while, usually after a course of medication or just with time. I learned that my attempt to control the outcome was fruitless, that to dwell on my losses was a way to avoid the deep sadness I felt. Trying to control the illness just stopped me from relaxing and accepting this new reality. As I let go of control in my mind, I discovered that I let go of tension in my body. To fight my body only served to expend the little energy that I had, and turned into fighting and blaming myself, just when I needed kindness. I came to believe in God or Spirit or Love or whatever, to have faith in some energy greater than myself that might help me cope with what I had been dealt. Perhaps if I couldn't control the physical effects of MS, I could have some control over how I responded to the illness.

Don't think that I've figured it all out, though. While I advocate the benefits of letting go, I don't always succeed. It can be hard for me to trust that events will turn out well. For example, I was pessimistic at times when we built our cohousing community, a close-knit neighborhood that was planned and now is managed by its residents. It took so long for things to fall into place — the money, the design, the building permits, the construction — that I used pessimism to protect myself from disappointment if the project was unsuccessful. "This will never happen," I'd say to my would-be neighbors whose homes were already completed while the building of ours was delayed. "Yes, it will," they would respond with optimism. "Just wait and see." And here we live now, with twenty-three other families who know and care about each other.

I wonder if the challenge with that project was to let go of the behavior of others — my neighbors, the bankers, the town officials, the builders. With MS, on the other hand, it is clear to me that I have to relinquish the mystery in my body. No one, not even my physicians, can make accurate predictions.

I'm fortunate that my MS has been relatively stable for the last fifteen years. I have come to call it "my MS," because it is an illness that varies considerably from person to person, and I have developed a relationship with that illness; sometimes it is one of anger or fear, sometimes one of peace. Flare-ups occur less often than they once did, but fatigue comes more readily. I know one day I may have a flare-up that could cause a rapid downhill progression. People ask me how I live with that knowledge. I don't really know. It's just my life. I've had to learn to let go in order to live well.

As I was writing this essay, I picked up a new book, *Learning to Fall*, by Philip Simmons. In it, Simmons writes about his search for peace after being diagnosed with Lou Gehrig's disease at age thirty-five. Imagine my surprise when I read in his foreword that letting go is the focal theme of the book. "When we learn to fall," Simmons writes, "we learn that only by letting go our grip of all that we ordinarily find most precious — our achievements, our plans, our loved ones, our very selves — can we find, ultimately, the most profound freedom." Letting go matters. It enables us to accept our losses and vulnerabilities and let in the unknown that is life's mystery.

Now, I am again challenged. Someone very dear to me will soon donate one of his kidneys to a close friend who is in kidney failure and on dialysis. It stirs me to let go and trust, in this case, that the transplant and recovery will be a success. There is some relief in knowing that I don't have the power to control the outcome. There is some peace in believing that an intangible source of life and love and optimism has influence, if only on my mental state. When I let go, I do know what I believe.

Childfree in the Suburbs
July 2002

Some of you feel sorry for me. Some of you think I'm selfish. Some of you think I just don't get it. Call me selfish, but I do get it. That's why I decided not to have kids. I get that children demand time, energy, and undivided attention. Fatigue from MS and its demands to pace myself forced me to think long and hard about having children. And I chose to be child-free. I prefer that phrase to "childless"; the latter denotes a lack, a less-than quality. It captures the loss, not the gain.

I don't want pity. My husband and I live in a close-knit neighborhood where we have children in our lives in a way that makes sense for us. Borrow and return. We have time and attention for one another that we don't take for granted.

Sure, I've had loss and longing. Loss of the possibility of a deep, continuous bond with a growing young person. Moments of longing for my own child. I am unsure how much of that longing has been for a child to nurture and cherish, and how much has been for the desire to fit into our culture of soccer fields and schoolyards, and to be fully admitted into the society of women. Growing up, my friends always knew they wanted children; I was never sure. Now, there is a club to which I do not belong.

Last year, my husband and I went to Provincetown, on Cape Cod, for a few days. We walked down Commercial Street, into art galleries. When there was a public walkway to the bay, we went down to gaze at the water and stroll on the beach, where the tide had not yet taken away the sand. We love to people-watch. One morning, I saw a man adjust the straps of a baby carrier that hugged a woman's body. I looked again.

Cradled inside was not a sleeping baby, but a terrier puppy. His four black and white paws dangled out of the canvas carrier.

The woman looked up at me and smiled. I smiled back and said, "That's wonderful!" "Yes, the dog sure thinks it is," she replied. At her direction, the man continued to tighten the straps until all seemed satisfied with the result. That puppy was as important to them as a human baby. As a child-free woman who adores her two loving cats, I knew the import of that moment. This club was open.

I asked my friend Nancy, during one of our walks in the woods, what she could learn from the child-free life. She quickly identified her own concern. "How will I find meaning once Lea leaves home?" she questioned. She wondered if that meaning could be replaced, if her work as an educator could fulfill her. "How do you find purpose?" she asked. "On walks like these," I replied. "Connecting with nature, connecting in relationship, as a pet-owner, a neighbor, a friend, a wife, a psychotherapist." Nancy's role as mother can never be replaced; it will only change while her life continues to have meaning.

I still remember a time, seven years ago, when I felt a deep connection with my then seven-year-old niece, Lili. We were at the unveiling ceremony of our Aunt Billy's tombstone. Billy had died a year earlier from lung cancer. Lili had told me that she didn't want to attend the unveiling, that she was scared. "I know," I replied. "It can be scary, and sad. We'll all be there together." During the ceremony, I was surprised when Lili left her mother's side and came up to me. She held my hand while she cried softly. "Why did she have to die?" she murmured. Her cries turned to sobs and she buried her head in my dress. I put my arms around her. It was the first time that she had come to me for comfort, instead of to her parents. Maybe she needed to maintain a connection to another aunt, to someone who could love her and let go a little more easily than a parent could of their child's pain. As I cried with her, I felt a mixture of sadness and love that defined the moment.

Judith Viorst writes in *Necessary Losses*, a timeless book from 1986, "Losses are a part of life — universal, unavoidable, inexorable. And these losses are necessary, because we grow by losing and leaving and letting go." Loss and longing are a part of all of us. How we each make sense of them is what matters.

Appreciating Life at an Uncertain Age
December 2002

Life is changing in some new and uncomfortable ways for many of us. It's called mid-life.

Memory is one of the many things we take for granted and then start to miss. I stand in the file room at work, trying to remember what I came to get. My friends and I write things down before we forget them. We keep a notebook beside the bed, in the kitchen, and in the car for just that purpose.

My sister-in-law reflects on her shifts in memory. Pat makes a phone call and then suddenly finds herself hoping that the person she's called will identify herself when she picks up the phone. My friend Marcia, similarly forgets the name of a friend standing before her. How many of us have experienced these instances of mortification when we can't remember who we have called or can't put a name to a face?

Those of us who have watched a parent disappear inside the vortex of Alzheimer's disease have a heightened fear of that shadow. I begin to read about perimenopause and am relieved to learn that hormonal changes can affect my memory.

We go backwards in time. My childhood friend Judy observes that she has begun to misplace objects like she did as a youngster. But now it's not her schoolbook or lunchbox that she can't find, but her pocketbook or reading glasses. Mid-life places us in a time warp.

We are adolescents all over again. The existential questions that faced us as teenagers have returned. What is the meaning of life and what is my purpose? I talk with other women about our place in the world, as children leave home and we reevaluate careers. Like teens, our bodies and moods are changing with fluctuating hormones. We no longer have the excitement of our first menstrual cycle, but the relief of our last.

When I was twenty-five years old and newly diagnosed with multiple sclerosis, I started to need naps and feel unusual sensations and pains. The illness set me apart from my peers. A doctor suggested that when I reached my late forties, I would not feel so different. Some of my losses from MS would mimic normal changes for my friends. I do feel an equalizing element with my peers now. Few of us pull all-nighters anymore or even stay out very late. I am no longer so alone.

Loss becomes more familiar. A child leaves home, we lose a job, a friend becomes ill, or a parent dies. We redefine our priorities and ask ourselves what really matters. Is it my accomplishments at work or my connections with friends and family that give my life import? We accept our personality quirks and learn to laugh at ourselves. We feel a new urgency to pursue our dreams. We still have time, but we now know it is finite.

Vanity goes out the window. When I was a teenager, friends whispered behind my back about my bushy eyebrows. "Her eyebrows are so big," I heard them say, to my horror. I felt embarrassed and ashamed that I couldn't control my changing body. I now know that they felt the same about theirs. For the last thirty years, I have plucked my thick eyebrows. But now, vision loss means that I can't see so finely. If I can't see those small hairs, then maybe they're not so important to hide. I let go of that vanity.

Eight years ago, a beautician remarked that she could hide the gray in my hair. But I hardly noticed the gray and liked what little I saw. I never returned to her salon again. After that episode, I asked my eight-year-old niece what color hair I had. Lili responded simply, "Black and white." Her matter-of-fact manner reminded me that appearance is in the eye of the beholder. Do we hide our age and exalt youth or do we accept these natural changes and live our lives fully? I wonder if it is time to accept myself, gray hair and all.

I ask my husband what signs of aging he notices in himself. "It's the hair that grows in the oddest places. My nose, my ears!" He remarks that people don't talk easily about these changes. "When we speak about them, we acknowledge our vulnerability."

At this uncertain age, we have become more vulnerable to loss and more susceptible to aches and pains. We take stock of our lives. Maybe it's time to let down our guard and pursue those dreams.

The Circle Remains Unbroken
May 2002

Asking for help can be part of the process of letting go. Last month, my husband and I spent a week in Chicago, assisting his parents while his mother recuperated from arthroscopic knee surgery. In her eighty-fifth year, Peggy's knee had begun to "lock," and decayed cartilage was the culprit. Surgery would scrape away the torn cartilage and return Peggy to health. Jim's dad is a historian, but not a cook, so Jim and I offered to come and help shop, prepare meals, and generally assist where we could. Although we weren't sure how Peggy would respond to this offer from her son and daughter-in-law, she was delighted by the prospect. Maybe after eighty-four years, pride in one's body is no longer a foundation of self-esteem. Accepting help can more easily be seen as a collaborative process of giving and receiving between people, rather than as a "weak," dependent state.

Living with MS for twenty years, I have learned to ask for help. This is difficult in a culture that places a high premium on independence. I have asked people to carry groceries for me when I don't have the strength, or to excuse me from an activity or a responsibility when fatigue dominates. To ask for and accept help has been a way to take care of myself. I've learned that people *like* giving; it strengthens the bonds of friendship. Now, I looked forward to helping someone else with physical limitations.

Peggy was delighted by our presence during her healing. She is generally an active woman, a daily swimmer and a volunteer researcher for the Oriental Institute of the University of Chicago. She was pleased to have helpful guests in her home who also spent time as urban tourists.

It was an easy week. Jim and I prepared our favorite dishes, ran errands, and had a delightful time in Chicago. We enjoyed the city's splendid lakefront and architecture. Jim's parents sent us off with their opera tickets on the day of Peggy's surgery. It felt wonderful to help, rewarding to witness how simple acts could mean so much to a woman who has done the same for so many. In my own life, I have experienced the vulnerability to illness and injury and how it brings an intimacy between people. I can trust others to see me in a disheveled state, far from the "together" person that I have let them know. I needed to experience the benefits of giving and feel the intimacy from the other side. Peggy let me in.

Sometimes emotional support is the help that's needed. When I was in graduate school in 1985, I had a flare-up of MS and overwhelming fatigue kept me in bed for three weeks. I remember a friend and classmate who called me every day to ask how I was and then just listened while I told her. She didn't demand anything of me; she helped me to scream, to cry, or even to laugh. I shed my facade and exposed my frailties, my rawness. I worried about how my vulnerability might affect our friendship, but Emily and I drew closer, not apart. It was the hardest thing I had ever done.

We live in a society that harbors a "myth of independence," a myth that autonomy and doing for self should be the aim of our lives. We view it as "weak" to ask for help; it threatens our identity. When ill, help may be more necessary and the vulnerability that much more intense. We may feel ashamed, that we are somehow less than others. But paradoxically, to ask for and accept help is a strength that promotes the qualities we associate with independence: well-being, resourcefulness, and initiative.

It is not always easy to depend on and trust in others. But it is interdependence that brings deeper human connection. I live in a close-knit neighborhood where we often exchange favors, whether we're ill or well. If Sue asks me for help with child care and I ask Kate for a ride and Kate asks Jim to assist with her computer, aren't we all giving and receiving from each other? The circle remains unbroken.

At age eighty-five or thirty-five, we are no less of a person when in need. In fact, it is the vulnerability that we humans share that connects us to one another. When we go deeper to those raw parts of ourselves, we can broaden our understanding of what it means to be human. I hope we don't all wait until disability or illness forces us to go on that journey.

Birth and Death on the Witch Hazel
April 2001

The witch hazel outside my front door has a sweet smell. I notice this as I walk by. Until just recently, snow sat on the ground by its side. Now, dead, brown leaves continue to hang on to its branches. It's an ugly thing, says my neighbor Caryn, who has one in her yard, too. But when I look closely at the bush's developing buds, I smell their sweet scent. I can just make out the crimson hue of the young buds, which are almost hidden by the dead leaves. There is birth and death on the witch hazel.

The oak tree on this side of the house — the shady side — demonstrates the same juxtaposition. Right now, dead leaves hang on there, as they have since last November. But one day soon, new buds will break forth, pushing off the old leaves. Some morning, I will notice that all of the dead leaves are gone. Life will win out.

I am fascinated by this process of the old dying and the new being born at the same time. It is ubiquitous. We know it happens to human life, all over the world, every instant. That the oak tree and this bush hold on to its leaves till the new are ready to thrive on their own is perfect. The natural world knows its order. Blossoms speak to us of what is possible. These dying leaves are not ugly to me anymore.

I am reminded of parents who hold on to their child's first bicycle while teaching that child to ride. And that final moment when the adult lets go of the bike. Possibility and wonder and power for the child. Loss and hope and possibility for the adult.

There is a different, yet similar, loss and hope when a client walks out my office door at the end of a psychotherapy session.

She has begun to say good-bye to the old, a body that no longer functions as it once did. Her tears speak to me of the loss. It is a life with illness that challenges her identity. She tries to adapt to the new, renegotiating a different path for herself in the world. She advances slowly, two steps forward and one step back. She may never be the athlete she once was, but she can create a life of meaning. She can bud again with possibility.

As the healing process is a test of faith, so, too, is this time of year. I don't have much confidence in early spring, with threats of snow still in the forecast. But by late April, my pessimism usually fades and again, I'm a believer. Crocuses are the first to stand up and be counted. I notice them in my neighbors' yards on my morning walks. They all say to me, "See, we won't let you forget. You can always count on us!"

Spring is about trust. Trust that the snow will melt and not return for six months. Trust that the trees will bear new leaves, that the daffodils will bloom to look like pinwheels, that the tulips will stand up tall and proud in their glorious colors.

Yet, it is this time of the year when I realize that I doubt the natural order of things. My trust is challenged, not yet confident that a hard winter is behind us. And I am not alone. Others comment to me that they, too, are still waiting. Some are wondering. The clerk where I go to purchase birdseed speaks to me with cynicism about the foot of snow in his back yard. I hear longing and doubt in his voice about its departure.

I'm told that the witch hazel held on to its luscious fragrance all winter. I missed out on it, though. I didn't think anything lived on my lawn then.

You Are Already There
June 2005

Driving home from Concord this afternoon with my husband, I feel that I am missing something. What did I leave behind? I touch my waist and locate my fanny pack. I touch my head and feel my baseball cap. But I still glance around the car and wonder what I'm missing. Ah, there's no fleece vest hugging my body, I realize. I don't need it. That's what feels so odd. The weather has changed. Finally. I don't want or need those extra layers to weigh me down. It's almost ninety degrees outside.

It always happens so quickly each spring. Fifty degrees two weeks ago, and then yesterday, fourteen-year-old Ben tells me that we almost reached one hundred degrees. Turning. Turnings. As the weather turns, I witness changes in others and in myself. The young men and women in the neighborhood, whom I met as infants fifteen years ago, when I was first looking into cohousing, are now completing ninth grade. The pre-schoolers graduate from high school today. I still see Hannah, playing on the floor with her dollhouse in her home on School Street, while I baby-sit so her parents can attend a Planning Board hearing to witness the approval of permits to build our neighborhood. And Lily, who I still see in her house on Spruce Street, is playing with her Barbie dolls in a little girl's bedroom full of dolls. And Bennett, with his inquisitive face, stares up at me as his parents and I meet each other for the first time to explore this interesting community called "New View."

More turnings: My dear friend Kate turns fifty, one of many turnings for us 1955 babes. In impromptu fashion, Kate moves her celebration to the lake, out of the hot sun. And again, in impromptu fashion, many speak and honor Kate's ability to genuinely appreciate others, to care for the land, and to relish the outdoors, even if it means playing in quicksand. When Patricia tells us the story of how Kate jokingly dared her ten-year-old son to jump into quicksand somewhere in the New Hampshire woods, I wonder about its meanings and metaphors. Seize the moment.

I reflect on my own turnings. I've embraced the heat and humidity of the last week, weather that does not suit me. In six months, I will have lived fifty years, half with multiple sclerosis, half without. I reflect on the wellness I feel, something I could not have imagined two decades ago when I used an eye patch to compensate for double vision and a walker to give myself balance. I know those symptoms may return at any time, or there may be new losses, but I don't dwell on that. I also know that it is time for me to let go of the "what ifs," the "shoulds," even the insecurities and the anxieties of "not being there" — not being smart enough or not achieving enough. Someone recently told me, "You are already there," in response to my ache to reach some pinnacle of achievement, some stamp of approval. I've printed out "You are already there" in bold and it now hangs on my study wall.

So I search for those words adapted from Ecclesiastes, Pete Seeger's words from "Turn, Turn, Turn." They remind me of beginnings and endings — "a time to be born, a time to die," and of joys and sorrows — "a time to dance, a time to mourn." These times will return, even peace is "not too late." Some moments happen simultaneously. A child leaving home is "a time to gain" as she reaches out into the world, and "a time to lose" as we miss her innocence. These are bittersweet times.

The seasons return again and again, as do health and illness, as do our insecurities and our centered moments. We will bundle up in fleece again. But now, we delight in blue sky, lush flora, and the freedom of only a few layers. I've left behind those layers that I no longer need. But all too soon, I'll pick them up once more.

Aging Towards Perfection
October 2005

The post-summer rush is back. We're all trying to get back on schedule again. I leave work to shop for a neighborhood meal. In a few days, I will help to cook the first community or "common house" dinner of the new school year. Forty neighbors are expected for curried rice, tofu, and vegetables. I'm thinking about this shopping expedition, but I haven't yet cleared my head of work and my clients. Focus, Dana, I say to myself. One thing at a time. That's my "almost fifty" mantra.

At the supermarket, I stare at the bag of rice in my hand, dumbfounded. If I need thirty-six to forty-five cups of cooked rice for forty people and this bag lists twenty servings at a quarter cup per serving, how many bags do I buy? I have no idea. My head wants to explode. Whether it's aging, perimenopause, my multiple sclerosis, or a combination of all three, I can no longer hold multiple items in my head at once.

It's getting worse. Five years ago, it was just my memory that I was losing. Now it's my organizational skills that are fading. Maybe it's not me that's getting worse; it's society. Everything is too fast. Email, cell phones, fax machines, instant messaging, all at our fingertips and racing us towards the finish. And we expect ourselves to keep up the pace.

Focus, Dana. Back to your story.

I decide to check out the frozen mushrooms and return to the rice later. In the frozen section, I'm pleased to find organic mushrooms. More pleased to read their portions and servings: three servings at one cup per serving. That's more straightforward: three cups per bag. I need thirty-six cups, so I'll buy twelve bags. In my cart they go. My legs feel weak from standing too long, and I look around for a place in the store to sit. Nothing. My eyes, which are also beginning to tire, well up with tears of frustration. Despite the return of humidity, I know that the sidewalk outside may be my only respite. But I want those cool September breezes back. Now.

I abandon my grocery cart in an empty aisle, walk out the door, and plunk myself down on the sidewalk to rest in the shade. I pull out my pocket calculator and again try to master the rice amounts. I suddenly realize that I don't remember the correct proportion of dry rice to cooked rice. I throw down my calculator, paper, and pen, and lean back against the cement wall of the building, "I can't do it all," I cry out to myself. I close my eyes and breathe in deeply, trying to find a way out. Some moments of rest later, I decide to let go of perfection and just do well enough.

I know I'm not alone with these concerns about aging. My friend Nola tells me of her new pastime, Su Doku puzzles, that help her mind stay active and focused. I wonder if this new puzzle in our nation's newspapers is the creation of some baby-boomer. A few weeks ago, another friend of mine drove to New Jersey, only to find herself in Pennsylvania. I guess she was confused.

I return to the store and am glad to find my cart undisturbed. I ask a fellow shopper about dry to wet rice proportions, and she casually says, "Oh, one to two or one to three. Either often works." I grab a guesstimated amount of rice and nine sixteen-ounce packages of tofu. Ah, more ease. That's nine pounds of tofu. Just what the recipe calls for. I spot an empty check-out line and walk up to the cashier. "You're having a party," he says, eyeing my very full cart. "Just a neighborhood dinner for forty," I reply. "Wow. Nice of you to shop," he adds. "Or crazy," I say.

The dinner is a hit. It is only a few days later, when in the same store, I notice that the packages of tofu are really marked with a weight of fifteen ounces, not sixteen or one pound. But no one seemed to notice the missing ounces in their meal, including me. Letting go of perfection worked out. There's a lot you can learn on a shopping trip.

More Than Just Another Yard Sale
September 2001

It is a mild Saturday morning, unusually warm. I don't like it, having begun to appreciate the cool September air. But I remember that nothing is normal anymore.

At home, I turn on the radio and hear NPR host Scott Simon. He is walking through the ruins of the World Trade Center: Ground Zero. His comforting voice assuages my grief, but his words evoke the loss, the anguish, the devastation. Tears come to my eyes, again. I can't help but think of those who managed to escape in that first instant and of those who tried to escape through windows but fell to their deaths. I picture lower Manhattan — cordoned off, choked with smoke and dust, carnage everywhere. After ten days of media bombardment, I am both overwhelmed and captivated. The news makes me shiver, but I can't turn off the radio. I'm in pain. I'm freaked out that our great nation can't protect us. When a plane flies overhead now, I stop and listen.

I trudge downstairs to the basement and locate the bicycle that I have tried to unload at every yard sale in my neighborhood for the last five years and will try to again today. The sign from the last sale still hangs from its seat: "$5 or best offer." This bicycle has traveled with me for the last fifteen years, but I haven't used it during all that time. I no longer ride due to loss of balance from multiple sclerosis, but keeping it has become a symbol of hope. And we do need hope today. At my neighbor Franny's suggestion, I change the sign, replacing "$5" with "25¢." Maybe this year the old bicycle will find a home.

When I arrive down the hill at the yard sale, I am surprised. There are more cars lining the road than I had expected. Perhaps our posted signs — "Yard Sale, 9/22, Proceeds to Red Cross" — have brought out more browsers than usual. I park my bicycle beside Franny's paraphernalia; she will oversee its sale. I say hello to David and his mother, who lives nearby in an assisted living facility. She is trying to sell things that she no longer has a home for. For a few minutes, I sit next to Pam, who is collecting money from purchases of used furniture, linens, toys, books, and more. A woman comes up to us with a bed sheet in hand and asks, "How much is this? I don't see a price." Pam decides a price on the spot. "A dollar," she states with confidence. The buyer gives Pam the money and says, "What a wonderful idea, giving all this to the Red Cross. It's more than just a yard sale." Yes, it is.

Today is also Acton Day, beginning at one o'clock, at the town's recreation area. Civic organizations will promote their purposes; children's activities will bring out families. During this last week, the town has decided to dedicate a memorial tree to the September 11 victims. I am determined to counteract my feelings of powerlessness and attend the planting.

My husband and I arrive early at the site for the scheduled event. There are only four others there. I am disappointed at the low turnout but realize the day's festivities have not yet begun. There is a maple sapling on the ground near us. I notice the orange and yellow leaves at its top and comment on their beauty. The woman next to me says the color indicates that the leaves are stressed.

There are now ten or fifteen people milling around the tree. A town selectman steps up to our group and begins to speak. He reminds us of the thousands whose lives were ripped away on September 11. We especially recall two town residents who were killed in the attacks. We know that any of us could have been there. Chills go up my spine. We are each invited to place a shovelful of dirt into the tree's hole. It is only a ritual; the burlap protecting the maple's roots will be removed and the tree planted later in the day. But today rituals are vital, for what else do we have?

I take my turn. The shovel feels solid; the dirt looks rich. I feel less helpless for a moment. I'm doing what I can, grieving with others. The hurt eases.

Jim and I return home. The yard sale is winding down. I see neighbors, cleaning up. I don't see my bicycle and ask if it was sold. "Two young boys bought it!" Franny exclaims. "They each donated twenty-five cents. They wanted to share it." "Terrific," I say. "How much money did we raise?" "Over $1,000," Franny replies. For the second time today, the pain lifts. I smile, with tears in my eyes.

NATURE NURTURES

The Tracks Left Behind
January 2001

Tracking an animal is opening the door to the life of that animal.... Our encounter with nature is largely a matter of seeing, and it relates to the quality of attention in our lives.

— Paul Rezendes, *Tracking and the Art of Seeing*

My forty-fifth birthday arrived with a whimper. I usually feel festive on these annual occasions, but I had pondered the coming of forty-five for too long. Close to fifty, half my life, no longer a child (oh, yes, I still am!), afraid that my life as a therapist, writer, and friend might become stagnant. Many of you know such feelings. So what was I to do?

I had a date that day to take a walk in our town's conservation land by Guggins Brook with my good friend Kate. I knew that I could feel silly, happy, or sad with her, and that something new and different was in store for me. Kate studies tracking, the art of reading animal tracks and signs as they guide us on the animal's path through the world. She shared with me the writings of Paul Rezendes, a tracker who explains that this journey is primarily a matter of seeing and teaches us how to pay attention to our own existence. It seemed meditative, a chance to notice my surroundings, listen to the silence, and recognize the natural world.

Kate and I began our trek in buoyant spirits, she with her eyes peeled for animal signs, me with my cane for added support. Despite my dismay at the number forty-five, I was delighted to take a walk in the woods. I talked about the day's significance for me. "Kate, this is truly a marker. Nineteen years ago this week, I was diagnosed with multiple sclerosis. I didn't think then of two decades down the road; that was too scary. If I had, I don't imagine that I would have envisioned feeling this well. I guess I have something to celebrate today."

We walked past the stone wall that marks the informal boundary between our cohousing community and the conservation land. We turned left onto the path that runs by the brook and noticed the ice that had formed there. I liked the cold of this day, though I didn't mind if the sun peeked out occasionally. Kate soon began to point out animal scat on the ground. She spoke softly, but with enthusiasm. "We saw pheasant scat here the other day! And yesterday, we saw fisher tracks on the ice. Animal signs are easy to find if you pay attention." To me, it just looked like poop. But Kate's excitement was catching, and I began to respect that these animals called this home.

We made a right turn, away from the brook, and followed a path into the woods. After a short distance, Kate grabbed my arm and said softly, "Look at this." She pointed to markings on a tree. "That's an antler rub. And here, where the deer have pawed the ground, is probably a scrape." Slowly and quietly, I was learning what it meant to be in tune with the woods.

We entered a thicket of trees and both began to remember the owl prowl that we took a few years ago with a naturalist from Drumlin Farm, a wildlife sanctuary nearby. We stood still and stared upwards at the top of a stand of white pine. I wondered if there was a creature silently watching us.

Kate described some of our furry neighbors' mating habits, how the scent of male urine in the snow or on a tree is designed to attract females, or how a female will rub herself against a tree to mark her territory and availability. I understood more clearly now my yet-unspayed cat's behavior while in heat. When she rolled on the floor or lifted her rump in the air, she comforted herself and called out for a mate.

Students of tracking believe that as we better understand the life of the animal, we more fully understand ourselves. Our closeness to nature helps us be sensitive to our surroundings. We attend to and care for life, and come to know ourselves in the process.

This world in the woods was subtle and quiet, yet evolving and alive. There was the running brook, despite the ice, the animal tracks that went one way and then another, birds swooping from branch to branch, the flash of a rabbit in the distance. All I needed to do was pay attention to appreciate this.

And if I pause long enough to notice, I will recognize the imprint I make on the world in my quiet meanderings through life. I leave markings in my passage that others will discover.

Walking in Season
April 1999

Walking is my exercise of choice. I am not alone in this endeavor. I often see walkers, stepping out on the roads of our town or along its occasional suburban sidewalks. This time of year, walking is made special. The warmth of the sun, the sound of birds chirping, and the sight of flowering buds accompany me. They are reminders of what is possible.

When I first began walking, my husband, Jim, and I lived in Jamaica Plain in Boston. I fell in love with Jamaica Pond, taking my morning walk around this tranquil body of water. Willow trees lined the walkway, ducks floated effortlessly in the water, and walkers greeted each other with friendly nods of recognition.

I began walking in the springtime, almost ten years ago. I was experiencing a bout of insomnia, brought on by a flare-up of multiple sclerosis. After doctors suggested that daily exercise could improve my sleep, I followed their advice. There is nothing worse than insomnia. During those dark moments of the night, when everyone else is slumbering, the isolation of the insomniac brings on loneliness and panic. I turned to my walks as a soporific.

The walks brightened my days. My extreme fatigue and leg discomfort lessened. I was pleased that despite MS, I could enjoy exercise. After a few months, I began to greet one older couple whom I passed every morning at the pond, and they, likewise, welcomed me into the day. We walked in opposite directions, neither of us changing our routine. Occasionally, we would stop and chat with each other. By late summer, I had learned that he was a retired ophthalmologist from Beth Israel

Hospital in Boston and that they lived nearby in Brookline. They learned that I was a social worker and discovered I had MS when they asked why I used a cane.

On Sundays, Jim and I often followed our road and entered a woodsy neighborhood with rocky outcroppings of Roxbury puddingstone. One morning in October, we wandered into this neighborhood and gloried in the tree colors of red, yellow, and orange. On our way back home, I wondered how long we would remain in Jamaica Plain. We both loved the city and appreciated the natural surroundings that J.P., as it is familiarly called, offered. But we were beginning to yearn for more open space. Jim, in particular, longed for trees. As a child, he had traveled every summer from Chicago to northern New Hampshire, where, for three months, he was surrounded by aunts, uncles, and cousins. He frolicked in streams and climbed the Presidential Range of the White Mountains, first as a young child and then as a hut master for the Randolph Mountain Club. The steadfastness of the trees nurtured him.

Jim and I joined the New View cohousing community in January of 1991. When the group chose Acton as the Massachusetts town where we would build, its conservation land was a major attraction. Here, we were allowed to cluster our homes in exchange for keeping a considerable portion of the land in conservation. Our site had an expansive feel because we abutted the Guggins Brook conservation land. Jim's longed-for trees could hug our dining room windows.

Jim is now the town's land steward of the Guggins land; he watches over the trees and coordinates trail maintenance. Now, when we take walks in the woods, he brings along clippers to cut back the thorny brambles that intrude on the trail. He tackles the bittersweet that is strangling the trees. His love of the woods has come home full circle.

I, too, delight in those woods, but I continue to relish my morning walks on the pedestrian paths of our cohousing community, doing the neighborhood circuit. I see the leaves on our maples beginning to sprout. Pam is out walking her short-legged corgi, and Bill and Nola are heading to their cars to go off to write and teach. Becky and Carol wave to me as they drive off to the train station. Sometimes, Franny sticks her head out her kitchen window and in a cheery voice wishes me good morning. I pass each home, silently wishing its occupants a good day. I think of it as my chance to awaken the community. I'm told that parents know how to dress their children in the morning by the number of layers they see me wearing.

When people ask me if I miss Jamaica Pond, I say that of course I do, there's nothing quite like it. But my walks continue in Acton, surrounded by nature and my neighbors.

Walk on.

Home Again
August 1998

You can go home again. Last weekend I returned to my summer camp of thirty years ago, along with forty other women in mid-life. We sang the same songs, canoed up the same creek, slept in the same cabins, and used the same outhouses. "Hillsboro Camp is a campy camp, not a summer hotel," was the camp's motto, and we were proud of it.

At the reunion, we even ate the same food. I had looked forward to the fried peanut butter and jelly sandwiches all the previous week, imagining that buttery taste melting in my mouth. Sure enough, it was the menu for Saturday's lunch. Turkey with the works was the traditional fare for Saturday night's "banquet." Proud campers that we were, at morning and at night we all stood at attention for flag raising and lowering as was the camp custom. We shared memories of our adolescent escapades — of smoking cigarettes in the woods and of rendezvousing with the local boys across the lake. I renewed old friendships and created new ones. We shared pictures of children and pets. It was striking to me that a significant number of these women, including myself, had chosen to remain child-free. Perhaps alternative folk were drawn to Hillsboro, or perhaps this camp experience helped us to create more options in our lives. The weekend was joyous and it was fun.

Hillsboro is no longer a camp for girls but a "family" camp that ex-campers take over for the first weekend in August. I had my doubts about returning, but Elaine, called Molasses at camp, convinced me to make the trip. I was concerned about how I would feel among friends of long ago who knew me when my body was robust and ever ready to play a game of tennis, take up the stern on a canoe trip, or horseback ride on my favorite mare, Lady. Now, with multiple sclerosis for the last seventeen years, my athleticism is limited to walking. I am blessed with that. But pacing myself among a group of friends, never mind people whom I rarely see, is always a challenge and something I must pay careful attention to. As I grow older, I'm more willing and even eager to set priorities, and more ready to say no to activities that will wear me out. It is always difficult to be with people I haven't seen in some time. If they know about the MS, they will be concerned about my current status. If they don't know, we have some processing to do together. So it took extra energy and motivation for me to go to this reunion.

At the reunion, I particularly enjoyed my talks with Jenny, not someone I really knew thirty years ago, about serendipity and faith. And I enjoyed a six a.m. walk around the lake, also not something I did as a girl. When I awoke Sunday morning, feeling rested although it was only half past five, I immediately thought of taking that walk I had never tried. So when I heard Oatmeal and Ibby, Molasses's sisters, get out of bed for a walk themselves, I said good morning and joined them at the washstand. The two of them were off for a walk into town; I told them that I would attempt the lake. They wished me good luck, alerting me that it was a significant hike.

My cane and I started out on the dirt road that goes through camp and then away from it, staying to the left side of Peace Pond, known as "the lake" to us. It was a cool morning and the sun was rising. I remembered how happy I had been for my warm sleeping bag during the night. I passed the camp's "rec hall," recalling the numerous plays that had been performed there, ones that I had watched and ones I had acted in. There was my first year of camp when we young campers put on a re-creation of the counselors in their private shack, called the

"Keep Out," and I pretended to be Little Murph with a cigarette hanging out of my mouth and singing "Twist and Shout."

I continued my walk away from camp. Birds had begun chirping in accompaniment to the bullfrogs who always croaked. That and the silence of the lake were comforting companions. I noticed the birch trees and the ferns by the side of the road and remembered the campcraft lessons of old where I had learned all those ferns' names — interrupted, bracken, sensitive, hayseed, New York. I recalled campfires that taught me how easily birch bark burns. Put it in with some kindling and you have a ready-made fire.

My legs were feeling strong, as they often did first thing in the morning, and I was enjoying my solitude. Fresh New Hampshire air always invigorated me. After ten or fifteen minutes, I came upon a T-intersection at the end of this dirt road, a destination I did not recall. I guess we never used to stray very far from camp (unless we were seeking out boys). I could still see my breath in the cool morning air, and I was drawn to the sun streaming down onto the grass at the side of the road. I sat down, my body soaking up the warmth.

After a few minutes of restoration, I continued onto another dirt road, which presumably continued around the back of the lake. Woods surrounded me; I could no longer see any evidence of the lake. I passed some paths into the woods and wondered if one of them would take me to the lean-to, a nearby campsite where the younger campers slept on their overnight hike. Curious yet eager to continue my trek, I stayed on the road. I passed some open fields on my left; on the right was a rickety house with a sleeping dog in the yard. A sturdy farmhouse seemed to go with the open fields; hearing me, another dog started barking and came trotting down a driveway. The dog and I stared at each other, both of us cautious. When I approached the drive, I stopped. The road continued but a posted sign read "Dead End." I followed a right fork, trusting that the lake was somewhere behind all those trees and if I just walked in this rectangle, I would return back to camp.

This next road was deserted. Its sides were heavily wooded. I looked at my watch, which indicated it was seven o'clock, and determined that I would only begin to get nervous at half past seven if I hadn't seen familiar landmarks by then. I realized also that if I didn't show up for breakfast in the mess hall by eight o'clock, others would become concerned and begin to look for me. I continued on with some buoyancy that I was on an adventure and that I just might succeed. Soon I could see that the road met another T-intersection ahead of me and that it was asphalt. I thought it an excellent sign; this was probably the road that led directly to the camp's entrance. I saw a car pass by ahead and was grateful for this sign of civilization.

When I got to the asphalt road, I didn't recognize the name on the street sign. That didn't mean anything — I never knew its name — and I turned right to complete my rectangle. There was still no evidence of the lake, but I didn't really expect to see the small body of water. I began to hear the clanging of cowbells up ahead and soon passed another tumbledown house from which I heard voices. The bells became louder and I saw three brown-and-white spotted cows in the field next to the house. I continued and looking straight ahead, I thought I saw a building whose larger size indicated that it could be Hillsboro Camp's Manor House. Then I saw someone in dark shorts and a white top — Hillsboro's green and white colors, perhaps? — walking down the road towards me. The taste of success was in my mouth. As we came closer to each other, I recognized Janie Vogt. Janie and I were the same age and had gone through camp together. I had learned from her over dinner the night before that as the niece of our camp director, Toxie, Janie was forced to attend camp and at first resented it. But Hillsboro grew on her and her attachment to the quirky camp came to equal my own. I was thrilled to see her at this moment. I had indeed succeeded in my hike! My legs felt it and Janie's face proved it. The Manor House was clearly in view now. We exchanged warm good-mornings and I reported that I had just walked around the lake. Janie was surprised and pleased that I had completed the two-mile trip. She continued up the road and I returned to camp, gleeful at my success and glad to have contradicted any assumption that MS prohibited me from hardy exercise.

As I walked back to Fiddle Inn, my cabin for the weekend, the pine scent of the woods reminded me of how Hillsboro felt like home. Crossing the bridge over the creek, I ran my hand over every bump and curve of the pine log railing. As Molasses had said yesterday, it all seemed so familiar. It was like riding a bicycle. Some things you never forget.

Hillsboro had been a special place. It still was. I learned from other returning campers that I had not been alone in my longing to leave the chaos of family behind every summer and arrive at a place that offered the best parts of childhood. How we would sob at the end of camp, not wanting to leave the intense bonds of friendship behind!

Reunions are full of memories that bump against reality. For me, this one was also fraught with the fear of not fitting in, a fear that illness exaggerated. But that weekend, I learned that Hillsboro was home and that we could all go home again.

Hoodoos and Beauty: Beyond What Is Known
May 2004

In the photo, I am grinning and sitting tall on Nate, a chestnut gelding. He is walking at the edge of a trail, high above the canyon's bottom. Shades of red, orange, pink, yellow, and cream glitter off the rock spires behind us. We are about to begin a three-hour trail ride to the bottom of Bryce Canyon in southern Utah. Our leader, Sean, puts the camera away, remounts his horse, and leads us into a fairyland of form and color.

After a steep descent for ten minutes on switchbacks carved out of pink sandstone, Sean says, "You've made it down the steepest section. That's the worst of it. I thought I'd wait to tell you." We trail riders giggle nervously in response. There are seven of us — three couples and myself. I think I'm the most scared, but maybe that's because Jim, my husband, commented on my bravery before I set off. I've ridden a horse only once since being diagnosed with MS over twenty years ago. I worry that the heat will trigger my symptoms and that my balance is too compromised for trail riding. Jim has gone on a long hike, while I dare to test my limits. What was I thinking?

But all is different here, a most beautiful part of the world. Golden spires evoking human form — hoodoos — tower two thousand feet above us. In order to see the top of them, I need to roll my head back and look straight up. As I do, I feel protected — nothing bad can get past the hoodoos.

The magnificence of the canyon humbles me. I don't really matter in front of this towering rock, millions of years in the making from wind and water erosion. My only task is to relish the beauty. The canyon is truly awesome, far greater than myself and my fears. Sean tells us that the Native Americans believed the hoodoos were humans stopped in time. I do not doubt that for an instant.

Sean assures us as we travel down the switchbacks that the horses are trained to walk on the rim. "Only one or two have ever gone over the edge," he jests. Rationally, I know these rides are safe, but I've had to sign a waiver absolving the leaders from any responsibility. So right now I'm scared. But Sean's wry humor and the expansive view throughout the canyon with its captivating rock formations turn my fear into awe.

The rider in front of me, on Scrib, wears a cap, decorated with the stars and stripes. The cap becomes my talisman. This world is beyond what is known. The magnificence of the sparkling multi-colored rock and the golden hoodoo spires overwhelms me and tears come to my eyes.

"This turn is a tough one," Sean says. "Keep your eye on Scrib. He walks quite close to the edge, but probably won't slip off." I giggle and then close my eyes as Nate follows Scrib to the edge. I relax as I feel Nate turn stolidly and I pat him in thanks. I open my eyes and in the distant patch of shade, the red earth is white. Sean points out Bryce Glacier and I recognize snow. It feels like eighty-five degrees in the sun, but Utah's snows hang on.

All of a sudden, Nate begins to trot. It's in his nature to catch up with his mates. My stomach flip-flops as my rear end goes bounce, bounce, bounce on the horse. I'm pushed to the left side of the saddle. I hold on to the saddle's horn for dear life. Nate decides he is the correct distance behind Scrib and returns to a walk. I breathe a sigh of relief.

My fear of the heat has passed. With next to no humidity, the warm, dry air refreshes me and I let go of my concerns. I feel too wonderful to worry about anything. What can I hold onto besides faith in the midst of this beauty?

Bounce, bounce, bounce. Nate is off again. I tighten my grip on the horn and it steadies me again. Sean turns around and says, "On Nate, shift to the right in your saddle." I'm glad Sean is watching out for me.

Back home, I stare at the photo of Nate and me. I think of faith and I think of Sean. I wish there were always canyons and cowboys to help me through the scary parts.

A Magical Mystery Ride above Treeline
August 2001

The hut master read the forecast at seven a.m. on Wednesday, August 29: "The summits will be in the clouds this morning. Visibility, fifty feet. Wind gusts, thirty to fifty miles per hour. Temperatures in the forties. Wind chill factor, seven degrees. The valleys will be in and out of the clouds all day. Be careful out there."

Madison Hut, at 4,800 feet and above treeline, was full with fifty hikers. Outside the windows was a swirling mist. We knew that the oatmeal about to be served was essential. Hiking companions turned to one other to assess plans. Jean and her husband, whom we had met the night before, were ending five days of hiking in the White Mountains of New Hampshire to celebrate their thirty-third wedding anniversary. They decided to take the most direct trail down the mountain, the Valley Way. It was protected from the wind by dense trees.

I turned to my husband, Jim, as he passed a platter of scrambled eggs, and asked, "What will we do?" We had hiked up the sheltered Valley Way from our cottage on Tuesday, due to threats of thunderstorms. The forecast had predicted clearing today and we had hoped to hike down the Knife-edge, a sharp crest on a ridge of Mount Adams, above treeline. It afforded gorgeous views into King Ravine, a large glacial gulf cut into the slope of the mountain. After twenty years of multiple sclerosis, I hike in these mountains. Three times slower than anyone else, but I walk on. As much as I wished to experience the ravine, I recognized the weather might make it unsafe today.

Jim and I agreed to reassess in a couple of hours. We could walk the few tenths of a mile to the Knife-edge and turn back if necessary. I remembered the sign that greeted us when we began our hike yesterday: "STOP. The area ahead has the worst weather in America. Many have died here from exposure even in the summer.... Turn back now if the weather is bad."

At eight o'clock, after comparing notes with other hikers, Jim and I began to strip our beds in the large bunkroom we had shared with twenty-five others and gather our belongings. I glanced out the window and saw that the mist was beginning to lift. I felt buoyant and decided to take a walk around the hut to evaluate the wind and temperature. I told Jim I would return soon. Now I truly understood the reason for warnings to hikers about preparedness. I was glad to have put on my turtleneck, sweater, and fleece tunic with my leggings and pants, and even more pleased to have my hat and gloves. I remembered leaving Acton in ninety degree humidity the week before and laughing when I packed this outerwear. Laugh no more.

I grabbed my trekking sticks and went into the dining room. Hikers sat at tables, talking. Others were on their way out the door and into the elements. We exchanged wishes for a safe trip. I stepped outside and felt the cold air, pleasantly surprised that it seemed mild. But the wind blew and intimidated me as I navigated the boulders. One moment I would be in fog and could barely see beyond a few rocks in front of me, and the next I would look up and see the top of Mount Madison with blue sky above her. I felt like I was in Brigadoon, the mythical Scottish village that appeared out of the mist every hundred years. Magical, mysterious, and joyous.

My task accomplished, I went back inside to report to Jim. He was packing our knapsack, including trash. The hut crew's skit of a bride and groom who vowed to carry out their trash for life had taught us well. Their focus on care for the natural environment and for hikers enveloped us all.

At half past nine, Jim and I were ready to leave for the Knife-edge. Blue sky had been present for almost fifteen minutes. We thanked the hut crew and said our good-byes.

We moved in and out of the mist on the rocks. We reached the Knife-edge and looked down into a deep ravine of beauty. Wavy lines of green scrub and gray rock were carved into the ravine's slopes, forming a kaleidoscope of form and color. A hawk dove into the ravine, then lifted to the sky. I was mesmerized. I would take a long time traversing the boulders down the ridge, but every moment would be precious.

A Mountain of Possibility
September 2004

It was early September and my husband and I were hiking on the Ammonoosuc Ravine Trail to Lakes of the Clouds Hut in New Hampshire. It had been a beautiful climb — we had hiked along the ravine, rested by spectacular waterfalls, and crossed the stream many times. But my legs were sore and tired. The last two-tenths of a mile had been very steep. I had ignored the words in the trail guide, "this section can prove arduous to many hikers," but they had come back to haunt me. I had been crawling on all fours, my technique over boulders and ledges, while Jim carried my trekking sticks. I needed to be cautious here.

There was no way I could safely descend this trail. We had two clear and dry days to make this climb. If the forecast was accurate, we'd reach the summit of Mount Washington tomorrow and come down on the Cog Railway.

We had been hiking for almost seven hours. "I need to know how much further it is to the hut. Will you go on ahead and see?" I begged Jim. "Sure," he said. "I think we're close." Close — how many times had I heard that word from hikers descending this trail? With twenty-three years of multiple sclerosis, I'm a very slow hiker, needing more than twice the guidebook time. Close is a relative term.

Jim put our pack down and gave me a hug, saying he'd be back in ten minutes or less. I placed my trekking sticks aside, sat down on a flat rock, and watched Jim disappear up the trail. The scrub was smaller and more sparse here, a clear sign that we were almost above treeline. Jim had been hiking all his life and part of me knew we would be fine. But another part of me wasn't sure. Would we get to the hut before dark? The predicted clear and sunny day had turned cloudy, and light was beginning to fade. Now I was tired and scared. What was I trying to prove by challenging my body like this?

I ate an orange, needing its thirst-quenching juice. I cradled my knees to my chest and stared down at the valley far below where I could see the outlines of the base station of the Cog Railway, our starting point. As I hugged myself, I took in the mountains; their magnitude enveloped and calmed me.

After five minutes, I began to wonder if Jim had located the hut. Time passed slowly while my anxiety returned. I remembered a directive *not* to separate from one's trail partner. What if Jim became lost? Unlikely, but fear made me envision the worst. I recalled the plaque we had passed on the first half mile of the trail, the section of easy grades. It memorialized Herbert Judson Young, Dartmouth '32, who had died there on December 1, 1928. Jim and I had imagined he got caught in a snowstorm; we added a memory stone to the pile on the boulder. Now I began to imagine that I would get caught in the rain and dark.

Later, in my need to understand the hiker's urge, I would ask friends and relatives why they climbed. Guy would remark that climbing posed metaphors for life. Susan would want to gauge her fifty-five-year-old body. Many would relish the wonder of the treeline experience and its expansive views. They, too, would feel they held the whole world in their hands. Doug would send me a quote from *Into the Wild* by Jon Krakauer — "A challenge in which a successful outcome is assured isn't a challenge at all." Their words would help me understand what I had been doing on that trail.

Soon I heard Jim's excited voice, urging me to come see the hut. I scrambled upright and joined him on the trail. This time, in much less than a tenth of a mile and at five thousand feet, we arrived at the hut.

The next day would be the clearest I could have wished for. With Jim's arm as a railing, I traversed the mile and a half of boulders to reach the summit of Mount Washington. There, with tears in my eyes, I looked beyond to the other Presidential mountains of Clay, Jefferson, Madison, and Adams and received a touch of something so large — a world of possibility. Right then, I had no doubt that this climb had been worth it. But will I want to face those risks and fears again? The outcome is uncertain.

COMMUNITY AND CONNECTION

Love Letters
March 1993

By 1993, when we future residents of the New View cohousing community in Acton, Massachusetts, began co-designing our common house, I had lived with MS for twelve years. MS was a big deal but it was not a big deal. I had a loving husband and worked part-time as a psychotherapist. After ten years I had learned to live with the unpredictability of fatigue, double vision, and loss of strength in my legs and coordination in my hands. It was just my life. The illness had taught me that life was precious and that people mattered. Cohousing came naturally to me.

It's the weekend scheduled for common house "programming," our term for group brainstorming and design, and I'm in the middle of a major flare-up. I draft a heart-felt letter, which my husband reads to the group:

Dear New View:

I write this at 2 a.m. as my body, full of steroids, resists sleep. I'm very sorry not to be with you today. It's hard, but I've learned that I must listen to my body when it goes awry (but God knows, I fight it). I'm having a flare-up of MS, mostly sensory, with lots of pins and needles sensations in my feet, torso, and face. Fatigue comes and goes unpredictably. So I turn over my trust to the group and know that you will program a splendid common house.

I ask as you program the common house to keep in mind the needs of any of us who become disabled as we live and grow old together. Mobility impairments, whether they demand canes, crutches, or wheelchairs, necessitate some accommodations. This episode has reminded me of my need for an easy grade around the common house and ramp or chairlift accessibility inside.

It's scary to write this, to expose my vulnerabilities, but MS is a part of me and I am conscious that we are all only temporarily able-bodied, though hopefully for a long time. I want our community to model a place where we can all live well with each other's love and support. I am so excited by what we are doing.

Lastly, I want you to know that I like to answer questions about my illness. It's a confusing and bizarre one. Pussyfoot around it, if you wish, but I prefer more than that. Everyone in my life deals with this added dimension in the way that fits for him or her. It's a process. Jim and I have coined a phrase for hard times with MS: "Just like life, only more so." We reset priorities, learn what's truly important, and understand our limits as human beings.

I thank all of you whose thoughts and/or words have been with me. I love you and am with you in spirit.

Love, Dana

My letter speaks of healing. Healing as care, not cure, as emotional, not physical. I am hesitant to write about the healing benefits of community, because I don't want to be misunderstood. I have come to believe that there are aspects of physical illness that we cannot control, that have a life of their own. I go to bed feeling well, and overnight my limbs become heavy, stiff, and tight. The reverse also happens. But I can control how I respond to and cope with the illness.

We blame the victim when we hold out certain models of cure — if she only had a healthy diet, did more yoga, saw that acupuncturist, had more friends. Well, maybe her tumor would have grown anyway, or he would have needed a wheelchair after the last flare-up, nonetheless. It is models of care, not cure, that the life of community offers. Care for the hearts and souls of its members, whether ill or well. Community and connection make a huge difference in the quality of our lives.

A week or so later, I am feeling a little better, and because I had shared my personal challenges with the group, I was determined to make it to the last programming session. I lie on my portable cot for most of the day, which enables me to participate. Afterwards, I write the community another letter, this time one of gratitude:

Dear New View:

I'm writing this on Saturday evening after programming. My heart is so full of your love and caring. I want you all to know how special and healing today was for me. That I could be with you in the way that I needed and that you could give me your hugs, love, tenderness, and caring is a tremendous gift.

The last few weeks have been tough for me. MS is more of an emotional battle than a physical one for individuals with this bizarre illness. When I feel isolated and strange in my body during these times, I so often feel isolated from people. I didn't feel that today. So many of you were just there, accepting me. I'm blessed that I can receive that, and we are all blessed to have each other.

Thank you for your healing energy, for help in lifting my spirits.
With love, Dana

Life, Love, Laughter, and Mud in Massachusetts
November 1995

"There's mud in my basement," Martha tells me. Martha and I are among twenty-four families building houses together, building a community of our dreams in which to raise children together and to grow old together, and there is mud in her basement.

It is a muddy process to become developers. What we've really wanted all along is to become neighbors and live in partnership — to play and laugh together, to fight together, to cook and eat together, to be with one another through good times and bad, to remain connected in a world that is linked by fax machines and modems and email but where the nuances of human connection have sometimes been forgotten.

Martha tells me that all seemed to be going well, that her family would move into their home in a month, despite the wrong cabinets, despite struggles with the building process, and now there is mud in the basement. My husband and I are involved in New View, as our cohousing community is called, to experience the support of community, a value I have come to honor, and to have children in our lives in a way that makes sense for us. When Kate and I visit our land to watch the building, her five-year old son, Ben, brings his baseball mitt. "Great," I say when they come to pick me up, "I'll get mine and we'll play ball." Kate later tells me that Ben exclaimed, "That is so cool! Dana has a baseball mitt." Having grown up with elders who showed me the joys of a good game of catch, I carry on that love with these children of our village.

Life is a muddy process at times. You slog through heavy soil and wonder if you will ever find smooth sand. That description captures some episodes I have had with multiple sclerosis for fourteen years, when for weeks my legs have felt weak and heavy as though I'm sinking in quicksand or plodding through mud, and then miraculously my body returns to myself and I'm again on solid ground. It describes another friend's struggle of experiencing the high joys in a new love relationship along with the fear and tension that accompanies such intimacy. My husband says that with such intimacy, we must be prepared to face the resurfacing of every issue we have. "Every issue," I hear, when we are in the throes of a disagreement that has brought us back to our child selves.

Decision-making has never been my strong suit. Yet that's what we must do, as my husband and I leave the community for a moment and focus on the design of our individual house. We have gone into a coffee shop, and the waitress asks us if we would like coffee, tea, decaf, or cappuccino and do we want it with regular milk, skim milk, soy milk, or black. Oh, and do we want a round table or a square table? "I just wanted coffee," I plead.

A member of a psychotherapy group I run asks me why there are group members who seem to have it all together. I tell her that all is not how it appears, that there are cracks under the finest surfaces. I remember a professor in graduate school who remarked about human misery to our class of budding social workers, "Everybody's got something," he said. "And if you don't have something, that's something."

And so we create New View to recover long-forgotten wishes and envision our dreams. It is not an easy task, wishing and dreaming in our building. We slog in the mud. We build the foundations of our lives. It is just like life, only more so.

Celebrate
Thanksgiving 1996

Thursday:

I wait with bated breath. Four households — nine adults and four children from our community — will join us on Sunday for a Thanksgiving meal. Since our common house at New View is not yet complete, there will be several community meals for us all to share in. Some will be for the vegetarians in the bunch; others will be for us carnivores. I will cook my first turkey. I feel like I am again in fourth grade, going off to Girl Scouts where Mrs. Rising will teach us the wonders of the culinary creation. But this time I am forty.

It is the coming-out party for the New View community. On Sunday, after the meals, a rock 'n' roll shebang will be held at Carol and Becky's house, where we will all put on a new face, a hidden face for some, and dance and sing our hearts out. And I will sing "Red Rubber Ball" at the top of my lungs in my black leggings and red blouse and with the sincerity that only a teenager can invoke. It may come the closest I ever get to my dream of a nightclub act. We are celebrating the completion of our cohousing community. All twenty-four homes are completed and occupied. I wait with bated breath.

Monday:

The turkey was delightful. I was out of bed and in the shower at eight o'clock on Sunday morning. With the excitement of an adolescent, I prepared for my coming-out party. I moved quietly, silently, so as not to awaken my husband. I dressed in my informal cooking and eating clothes and went into the kitchen to prepare the bird. It didn't make sense that I was leaving Jim in bed. It didn't make sense that I had a husband. I felt the tingling excitement of a child before her birthday party or before her first piano recital. But this time I was to sing.

First to the bird. My arm went into her cavity and pulled out her neck, kidneys, giblets, all wrapped in paper. Peel the onion, cut the celery, snip the parsley. And back into the cavity I went. It was almost nine o'clock and I could already bring the bird to her fate — the oven. "Am I a grown-up now?" I asked myself as I shut the oven door on that first turkey. Carol had created the stuffing, and she and Becky arrived at one o'clock to make the gravy. Other friends brought their essential ingredients. Martha and Bill donated cranberry sauce and sweet potatoes. Franny made her mom's favorite dish of Brussels sprouts and onions, and her husband, Bill, carried over extra chairs from their home next door.

The meal had a resplendent air, just as Thanksgiving should. We added extra leaves to our dining room table, which gave a banquet-like tone to the occasion. We set up a small, octagonal table, which delighted the children at our affair. Carol's daughter, visiting from Israel, brought her own food, which she could eat informally from their containers, allowing her to keep kosher. We reminisced about a Thanksgiving we had all shared some years back, before we had even found land to build on. We imagined a future Thanksgiving in our common house when we could all dine with ease under one roof. We delighted in the opportunity that we have taken, without a common house, to really appreciate each other's homes. We feasted, trying to save room for dessert, which would be served later in the afternoon.

At three o'clock the community congregated at Becky and Carol's for the rock 'n' roll celebration. The highlight for me was no doubt my rendering of "Red Rubber Ball." Patricia, one of the few professional musicians in the bunch, backed me up on the piano; Eliot's bass guitar gave us depth, Jim's saxophone offered soul, and Sue's drumming set the rhythm. I belted out the song — "I should have known you'd bid me farewell. There's a lesson to be learned from this and I've learned it very well." And with the genuineness of a scorned lover, I continued, "Now I know you're not the only starfish in the sea. If I never hear your name again, it's all the same to me." Patricia's full and experienced voice joined me in harmony on the chorus, "And I think it's going to be all right. Yeh, the worst is over now. The morning sun is shining like a red rubber ball."

As I walked off the stage, which was only a living room but felt like much more, the cheers rang out. I received praise ranging from "Will you sing again?" to the report from Patricia that her son exclaimed during a break, "Mom, Dana was really good!" An acquaintance commented that she could tell I had some history there. Well, the song did bring me back to high school and college days, when I was led astray by myself and men whose interests were really elsewhere. With my unconscious anger along with my uncontrollable joy, I sang the song to all those men who jilt women as a hobby and dedicated it to all those women who live through difficult times before finding themselves.

Food continued to add warmth to the affair. Desserts brought by New View residents were laid out across Carol and Becky's kitchen counters. Brownies, cookies, tofu cheesecake, apple pies, pumpkin pies, orange slices, and more offered something to diners of all persuasions.

I am left with strong memories from the day: my first turkey, roasted brown and tender, Carol and Becky's house with a room full of New Viewers, a sudden realization of what we've accomplished, tears welling up in my eyes and a lump forming in my throat, and the thrill as Patricia gives that first drum roll and begins with "Start Me Up." Other girlfriends sing "Stop in the Name of Love." Young girls sing the back-up to yet more love songs. I am left with the realization that rock 'n' roll and frustrated love are synonymous. Larry sings a folk tune for New View in which he's altered the words of John Prine in order to tell our tale. My husband wears shades and a black top and pants. He is an amateur who plays his sax with extreme couth. We all rock 'n' roll.

The music ended at six. I had skipped my regular five o'clock nap, not wanting to leave and miss the fun. But I was fading. Jim and I came home, and I collapsed on the bed. The clock said half past six. I fell fast asleep until a quarter past eight and got back in bed for the night at half past ten. I dreamt of turkeys playing the sax.

The next day we returned to normal, back to work for the adults and school for the kids. My young neighbor Hannah came home sick in the middle of the school day with laryngitis. She said she had felt it coming on at the end of her last song but ignored it.

Monday evening:

In the evening Becky calls, looking for her red slippers, which she believes she left behind at our meal. I go down to return them and retrieve the red rubber ball, my prop, to return to Marcia. Jim comes along to get his jacket and sunglasses, left at Becky and Carol's home the day before. The community is putting itself back together again after the big bash.

Co-existing
Fall 1998

My eyes feel hollow. My head feels like a bowling ball. Throbbing. The sides of my face feel like someone has beaten me up. My legs are made of lead. I plod through my day. This isn't a new exacerbation; it's the recurring symptoms of multiple sclerosis. I remember the words of my first neurologist from seventeen years ago, "This, too, will pass." Her optimism calmed me then and I want it to now.

It is five o'clock. I lie down, in preparation for dinner at my neighbors' at six, a weekly event in our neighborhood. When I awake, the house is quiet. I call out for my husband. No response. Has he left for dinner? I turn and look at the clock. It says 6:46. I suddenly notice that I can move my head without fatigue. My body feels at peace. My body is my own, no longer trapped in a spider web of tight muscles and aching joints.

I get up and dress in a daze. I move slowly, not entirely trusting how well I feel. I call Marcia, ask if there is any dinner left. "Plenty," she says.

When I walk into her home, I see friends talking, laughing. Children are playing. My very young friend Sam sees me and grins. I tell myself that I will go over and give him a hug later. I want to yell, "Everyone, I'm okay. Come talk with me. I can engage with the world." Marcia interrupts my silent soliloquy as she gives me a hug and says, "Wait here. I'll get you a plate of food." I follow her into the kitchen where an array of Mexican food awaits. She puts two enchiladas on my plate, rice and beans. Marcia seems to know just what I need. She senses my feeling that I have just risen from the dead.

Neighbors and friends fill the living room and kitchen. I spot an empty seat at the dining room table and go there. I am amazed that my head and eyes are still clear. I smile for the first time in three days. My husband sees me from across the room, comes over and gives me a hug. "I'm okay. It's gone," I say to him with pleasure. He smiles.

The evening continues for me in a serene sort of way. I stay seated; friends come over to chat. They greet me with warm hugs and smiles. I feel their love. Did they know I was not feeling well? Later, I realize that it was I who projected love, feeling comfort with a body I can trust for now, with my ability to simply appreciate the warmth of friends. Sometimes in a life with an illness like MS that brings unpredictable hours of sensory puzzles and bodily fatigue, what matters most are the simple things — a child's laugh, the hug of a friend, the hearty taste of black beans.

One conversation I have that night is with my friend Sue. She learned the day before of her friend's death from breast cancer. She tells me, "I'm doing OK. I've cried. Things co-exist." She pauses and with tears in her eyes, repeats, "Things co-exist."

Yes, things co-exist, I think later, walking home with my husband. The memory of pain, knowing its tentacles are just around the corner, exists. And so does the soothing pleasure of the evening.

Play Ball!
March 2000

"See you soon," I say to Jim as he leaves the common house to go home. I sit on the bench to put on my boots and battle yet another New England snow. Aaron is sauntering by the stairs inside the common house. Many of us have just enjoyed a scrumptious brunch on this Saturday morning, lovingly prepared by our neighbors David and Pam. Bagels and eggs — scrambled for some, omelets for others, with fillings of onion, peppers, mushroom, or cheese — keep us satiated. But nine-year-old Aaron doesn't seem thrilled. Brunch food does not excite him. "Hey, Aaron, you look bored," I say. "Yeah...," he replies as he shuffles in the hallway. This brunch mostly attracts adults; Aaron is the lone child hanging around. His twin sisters are probably off somewhere, engaged in imaginative play.

Jim and I are child-free. Having children in our lives is one of the things that attracted us to cohousing. I will take advantage of this opportunity. Spontaneously I ask Aaron, "Want to go downstairs with me and play some Ping-Pong?" Aaron's face brightens and he says, "Yeah!" "Let's go play," I say emphatically. I put my boots aside and off we go.

"Are you any good?" Aaron asks me when we are down in the basement. I take off my sweater and we both pick up the paddles. "Not bad," I say, and I mean it, though I haven't played for many years. Oh, I hit the ball around recently when the new table was placed in the common house, but I haven't really played. I used to be fairly good at Ping-Pong, having played for hours as a youngster with my brother on our porch in the New York suburbs. But with poor coordination and unsteady legs from almost twenty years of multiple sclerosis, I can't guarantee my game anymore. But I still love the sport. I hope I'm not leading Aaron or myself astray with my words of assurance. I don't know if Aaron knows or understands about MS, but it doesn't seem to matter.

We spend a few minutes just hitting the ball to each other, checking to see if our games are compatible. My first shots are embarrassing. I either swing at the ball and miss completely or send it off the table without a bounce. I imagine that Aaron is wondering what he got himself into. Consistency isn't his strength, either, but he does wield a spin, sending me shots at times that are impossible to return. As I warm up, my game improves. Ping-Pong is like riding a bicycle. Some things you just never forget. My swift, low serve returns to me. Our rallies make it to only three or four shots over the net, before we have to chase after the ball, but I am enjoying myself. Aaron's bright countenance indicates that he is, too.

"Want to play a game?" Aaron asks. "Sure," I reply. "Just remind me of the rules." Aaron reviews these with me and we decide to play a game to twenty-one, alternating service after two serves. Aaron begins and wins his first two service points with ease as I miss the returns completely. My fast serve allows me to catch up and the game is tied. Relieved that Aaron won't slaughter me, I relax. He stays one or two points ahead throughout the game. I might get one point from my serve, but when Aaron returns with that spin, I am lost. Even my older brother hadn't learned that trick when he was nine. The game ends, twenty-one to nineteen, with a win for Aaron. We are indeed a good match and I ask Aaron if he is willing to try another. He says yes, and we agree to play this second game to just eleven. My stroke has found itself by this time, and I triumph at eleven to five, though I haven't managed to return any of his spins.

Needing to pace myself, due to fatigue from MS, I don't often engage in activities without thought and planning. But children and spontaneity came to me that morning. Although my legs feel sore and tired as I hobble home, I know my bed awaits me for a rest. When I enter our house, Jim is in his study at the computer. He turns to me and says, "You got involved in something." "I sure did," I reply. I give him a hug and tell him I have been reviving my spontaneity skills.

Volleyball Means Never Having to Say You're Sorry
August 2001

This summer, we play volleyball on Friday nights in my neighborhood. Steve set up a net last month and some of us have taken to the sport. I am thrilled with the idea, but am afraid that I won't fit in with the competition.

There is a game, of sorts, in progress tonight. Four of my neighbors are on each side of the net, and they hit the ball to one another, or "set" (tap) it to a teammate, or one player hits the ball twice in a row. I watch from the sidelines as petite Nancy serves, swatting the ball with surprising strength. I join in with cheers as the ball sails over the net. Linsey rushes to the ball for a return and runs into her dogs, Scooter and Luna, who are frolicking on the "court."

"Interference!" cries out my husband, Jim.

We all laugh; Linsey and her teenage son, Joey, remove the dogs from the game. There is real intention here, not to play by traditional rules or to score accurately, but most definitely to hit the ball and have some fun.

Sal calls out the score, "Eight, eight!" Ten-year-old Jake questions why the score is always tied. It doesn't seem correct. "Of course it is," says Sal.

I watch for a while this first night, thinking I might join in. I am cautious; the last time I played volleyball, I was twenty years younger, strong-legged and coordinated. But these are my friends, relaxed and having fun. And after all, I still play a decent game of Ping-Pong. I could belong.

"Join us," Nancy calls over to me, and I do.

Cooperation reigns. Rules are more like guidelines; scoring is secondary. Any strange play is allowed, if it makes the game more interesting. We welcome all ages and skill levels. We laugh, run, fall.

I do fit in, even without much of a game. I'm good at rotating when it's my team's turn to serve. If the ball comes near me, I run from it or look up and miss it entirely, becoming quite dizzy in the process. I connect with the ball once, and, to our delight, a teammate taps it over. When I rotate into the service position, Nancy hands me the ball and tells me to go for it. "It's been a long time," I call out in warning. But my body has memorized the motions. I hold the ball in the palm of my left hand, my right arm swings back, and I punch the ball with a closed fist. It goes into the net. "Redo serve, and move up a little," calls out Sal.

I try again and somehow the ball sails over the net. Cheers explode. The other side hits it out. I rub my wrist, which is smarting from the sharp service contact with the ball. "Yeah, we're all suffering," says Nancy, who stands next to me. "But it's worth it," I insist.

My next serve goes into the net. "Sorry," I say automatically. Linsey tells me that apologies are not allowed. "Volleyball means never having to say you're sorry," Jim adds, and we all laugh. We are putting the shame of childhood ball games behind us.

It is another Friday night, and Steve gives a clinic on how to set and serve. Nancy tells me she has finally learned to wait for the ball, not to jump. We comment on how much easier it is to learn without pressure. I tell her I may have played better twenty years ago, but it wasn't this much fun.

Becky is wearing a pair of black and brown gloves that look very official. I ask her where she got them. She says they were in her garage; they are volleyball gloves now. "Okay, you have the intimidation factor," I say. "I'm convinced you know what you're doing."

"Ha!" laughs Becky. She, too, then punches a solid serve. Steve, one of our experienced players, returns the ball gracefully, and my team manages to hit it back. Jim hits the ball on the other side, setting up Linsey, who hits it over.

Finally, a rally! Cheers erupt as we feel proud of our accomplishment. It feels like a real game is in progress. "A volleyball moment!" I exclaim.

It's getting dark and mosquitoes are on the rise. To our glee, Sal calls out a tie score. "Twenty, twenty. Next point wins the game." We all get that point.

Balancing Private and Public
March 2001

Martha, Kate, and I roam the narrow strip of woods by my house, trying to resolve the group's continuing conflict over the design of the woods path. I argue for a winding path of reduced grade to attend to the needs of people with disabilities, Kate wants to honor environmental concerns and save trees, and Martha wishes to respect the privacy of residents shielded by the woods. Some of us want all three, which heightens the tension.

"I'd be willing to lose some trees if they are closer to your house than mine," says Martha. "I might consider a six percent grade, rather than four percent, to save some trees," I return. "As long as we create a resting area where the path is steepest." And we do just that.

Now it's Monday of Presidents' Day weekend. I've been less social than usual these last three days, hanging out with my husband and our cats and holed up with a fine book, Barbara Kingsolver's *Prodigal Summer*. But it is time for dinner and I put the book down.

Dinner takes place a few times a week in our common house. This is the heart of our cohousing community, where people gather for meals, meetings, and parties. The common house was the most recent product of our ten years of working with two dozen other families to locate land, hire professionals, get permits and financing, and build our twenty-four house neighborhood on a hillside in Acton, Massachusetts.

Cohousing was named by two American architects inspired by communities like this in Denmark. There are now forty-six cohousing communities in the United States, and many more in the process of being created. Resident-designed and resident-controlled, cohousing has a pedestrian orientation to encourage spontaneous interaction. Cars are parked on the periphery. Walkways connect the homes. There is open space for safe play. All this appealed to me and my husband, who both value community. And although we have chosen to be child-free, we still wanted children in our lives.

We got to know and like our future neighbors in the process of working together as amateur developers, using consensus to make our decisions. We drifted apart from our neighbors a bit while the individual homes were being built and we all focused for many months on countertop designs and appliance selection and the best white wall paint colors for our individual homes. We came together again in the common house.

One challenge that the common house presents to each of us is the need to discover the balance between privacy and community. All of us can prefer the solitude of our own homes at times, and because MS fatigue can be exacerbated by sensory stimulation, I sometimes have mixed feelings about visits to the common house. I know I must pace myself when I go there. I return to this particular evening, six or seven years ago.

Although I have been in a solitary mood all day, or maybe because of this, I look forward to tonight's meal. Depending on the whim of our volunteer cooks, it's not unusual for there to be meat and vegetarian options at our dinners. Tonight, four-year-old Kaya and her mother, Sue, are to prepare pizza for the kids; Jim and Nola are making chicken stew and vegetarian chili for the adults. Kaya is standing behind several trays of pizza and greeting those of us who have signed up for this meal. Her head comes up just above the counter and she looks very official in her blue apron. I walk around the counter to kiss the top of her head and tell her she looks great. "Are you having fun, honey?"

She nods her head vigorously, but stays focused on the trays of pizza.

I move to the large pots of chicken and rice, whose aroma is making my stomach growl. After doling out a portion for myself, I notice the bowls of condiments for the chili — sour cream, yogurt, cheese, and cilantro. I nab some yogurt to go with my chicken. My husband and I look around and decide to sit at a table with Mary. She is talking excitedly with Jane about a successful day at her art studio, leading workshops for kids and parents. Mary is a retired French teacher, now an artist, whose creativity has inspired many in our community and beyond. At the age of seventy-two, she continues to embrace the child's joy and her own.

Martha and Bill are alone at a table next to us, talking intently. Their two boys, ages ten and four, are off playing somewhere. I know that these parents appreciate this time for conversation. Two drumming teachers live in the community. Some of their students will give a drumming recital after dinner. My book calls me home, though I am a bit wistful about leaving.

I sometimes worry that my need for "alone" time won't feel acceptable, living in a cohousing community. But on nights like this, I realize I can have my cake and eat it too. Tonight, my solitary spirit enjoys a visit to the warmth and camaraderie of friends in community.

PORTRAITS

A Crucial Choice
October 1999

I got out of my car on this damp and cold Saturday and noticed that the sun was trying to shine. Young boys, men almost, jostled with one another in the crowded parking lot. Cars lined the street in front of the Unitarian church. From a few blocks away, I had glimpsed the church and the row of cars. They had assured me I was headed in the right direction.

I entered the tall, white church, into the comforting familiarity of New England's own. I was struck by the large number of people here for the memorial service, but I was not really surprised. I knew no one, though I searched for familiar faces. Lucinda affected these lives, I thought. Her church had become a family that reached out to her and listened, that laughed and cried with her, that cared for her during these last weeks.

I had known Lucinda for only a few short months. I supported her in the struggle to come to terms with her life and illness. I was a witness to her choice to end the medical treatments that were sustaining her but not improving her quality of life.

I learned of her as a woman who had felt powerless when a young girl to stop the physical and sexual abuse that had surrounded and enveloped her. I saw a woman who had left that family and made her way to educate and support herself. She had battled severe depression and come through it. She had spoken publicly about abuse prevention.

A congenital disability called for surgery in her late thirties that required a blood transfusion. The blood was tainted with hepatitis C, and Lucinda was found to have these antibodies a few years later. Since she was not a candidate for a liver transplant because of her complicated medical history, Lucinda chose to live life as best she could. She shared her beautiful singing voice with the church and cultivated friendships with this new family.

When she joined our three-month psychotherapy group, she had not yet made the choice to die. With seven others who faced the challenge of living with illness, she voiced this solitary experience and gained comfort in knowing she was not alone. The illness had weakened her body and she endured greater limitations daily.

She spoke of loss. She had given up driving and her volunteer work as a foster-care reviewer. Letting go of the latter may have been the most difficult choice for Lucinda. Knowing the impact of a troubled childhood, she had tried to better the lives of children in need. "My life has become circumscribed," she said to me when I first met her. "It's a sense of loss I feel, not anger." In her more vulnerable moments, Lucinda wondered what she had done to deserve the series of traumas that had captured her life.

In the last month of the group, Lucinda spoke of her decision to end the frequent blood transfusions that were keeping her alive. She said she was afraid that this would be uncomfortable for others and impede their process of learning to live with their illness. I remember my thoughts and questions. Was this a suicidal act? Couldn't Lucinda continue to find meaning in her volunteer activities? She had informed us that coming weekly to group was one of the few activities towards which she chose to devote her energy. Had her stamina diminished more than I realized or accepted? Did I need to meet with Lucinda individually to assess whether a severe depression had returned and if this choice was her way to "act out?" What was my ethical responsibility?

Lucinda spoke clearly of the decision to die, one that she had thought deeply about and discussed with her minister, closest friends, and health-care providers. I began to recognize my discomfort with death and wondered if I wanted to "evaluate" my client as a way to hide my uneasiness.

Lucinda's ability to speak openly of her decision helped me and the group members to engage with her and voice our thoughts and feelings. It was a few weeks before I said those taboo words, "death" and "dying," in Lucinda's presence. But once I finally owned the reality of what was happening, it eased our anxiety and helped us talk about our inner experience to Lucinda and ourselves. I wanted this to be a healing process for the group, to recognize their feelings about Lucinda's decision and to say good-bye with her. Members shared feelings of sadness and understanding. A few questioned her choice, wondering if she had other medical options. Maybe some felt angry but were unable or chose not to voice this emotion. Lucinda patiently told us that she felt this was the right decision for her.

I wondered afterwards to what extent Lucinda had considered the choice to die before joining the short-term group. I questioned if I had failed, ethically or therapeutically, to fully explore her decision. Had I done enough? Once she spoke of it in group, she had clearly chosen. There were others with whom she had processed this option, medically and spiritually. She had looked to this group of peers to witness and validate her illness experience; it was a genuine connection with others who knew life with a chronic illness that Lucinda had sought and received. She had not used us to help make the choice to die but to truly understand the marginality that she felt. Perhaps she needed that bond in order to let go.

Lucinda showed us the empowering role of choice. She wanted to take charge of the end of her life, not suffer unnecessarily. It's not a choice to wish on anyone, but to stay centered as she did and to continue to extend herself to those around her, not withdraw as many do towards the end of life, reflected the best part of Lucinda. And this allowed the group members and myself to ponder those best parts of ourselves that we too often keep hidden.

I never did meet alone with Lucinda. I have some regrets about that choice. Maybe it would have made me feel better about her death if I was convinced I had done my job more thoroughly. But I don't think it would have changed the outcome of her life.

The final anthem of the memorial service, a service that Lucinda had designed, was Robert Frost's "The Road Not Taken," set to music by Virgil Thompson. I thought of the road that Lucinda had not taken and the one she followed. She chose a dying and a death that was full of love and care, the kind of life that she had wished for herself and others. It was a gift she could bestow on herself and on all of us. Thank you and good-bye, Lucinda.

Walking on the Border
November 2003

I was on the other side, the side of health. I was not the patient in need. My brother-in-law, Bruce, was in the hospital with atrial fibrillations, too rapid heartbeats. We waited for doctors to figure out the correct combination of drugs to stabilize him.

My husband and I visited Bruce at the Boston hospital, known for its excellent cardiac care. It was different, being on this side. I wanted to fix things for Bruce. I didn't like seeing a loved one in the hospital, monitored by wires. I felt a stabbing powerlessness; this illness was not in my body. At least with multiple sclerosis, I knew what I experienced: the fatigue and the weakness, the eye and facial pain, the numbness and tingling, the difficulty walking. I had learned to ask for help. After twenty-two years, my MS had a predictability, for now. I had not had any new MS symptoms for several years, but I was accustomed to walking on the border of illness and health. That was not Bruce's role in the family. Wouldn't it make more sense if I were the one in that hospital bed?

Bruce spoke about the frustrations of hospital life — the waiting, the errors with meals he'd ordered. But he had good coping skills for a hospital stay. He related well to the nurses and other patients. He asked questions and stayed informed about his progress. He learned about the surgery that could treat his condition if medication was not a long-term solution.

Bruce began to feel his heart racing and looked at the monitor. Sure enough, his heart rate was now twice as fast as it had been a few seconds before. Bruce was a healthy man, despite these heart irregularities. He wanted to go home, but not until this was under control. He was bored at the hospital, but unwilling to leave its twenty-four-hour care. He told us that until the medication kicked in and his heartbeat had stabilized for a few days, the risk of blood clots and stroke remained. I thought then how we are all so close to the other side of sickness or health.

There was nothing I could do but be a friend on this side. How helpless Bruce must have felt! And my sister, Trinka, waiting at home when she wasn't working or visiting Bruce. His condition was not life-threatening, but the risks were severe. Bruce was walking, talking, even doing a little business by phone. His disorder was acute, not chronic. I noted the differences from multiple sclerosis. MS symptoms rarely demanded an urgent response. The risk of stroke or death was unusual. Yet surgery couldn't cure MS.

We visited with Bruce for forty-five minutes. A volunteer delivered flowers from Bruce's colleagues; friends and family called. We talked about sports, Thanksgiving, and loss of control. An orderly arrived to wheel Bruce off to an examination by a pulmonary specialist. Jim and I went out for lunch and then returned when Bruce did. We stayed for another hour. I didn't want to leave.

A few days later, I received an email from Trinka. She thought that Bruce would come home soon. Could we host Thanksgiving, instead of my mother in upstate New York, so Bruce could stay close to home? My mother would come to the Boston area early and cook. My brother and his family would drive up from New York. I so wanted to give to Bruce and my sister. My family had often accommodated my needs due to MS. I had been feeling well and wanted to give back. I conferred with my husband, and we readily agreed to offer our home. I called Trinka. "We're happy to host Thanksgiving," I said. "I want to."

Bruce soon came home and our Thanksgiving was splendid. My mother's food — stuffing, squash casserole, string beans with almonds, and chocolate roll cake — was delectable. My turkey, moist and tender, melted in our mouths. The eleven of us went around the table, each offering our thanks — for Bruce's health, my health, and our mother's lively presence.

I discovered some things from Bruce's ordeal, about myself and illness. I felt envy for the attention that Bruce received. My sick persona was lost. My feelings jarred me — as does change, with its unpredictability. I don't dwell on how my MS could get better or worse at any time without warning. I like the illusion of stability. Bruce's sudden trip to the land of the ill and back reminded me starkly that stability is ephemeral. What is lasting is our connection — our ability to reach out and ask for and offer help — across the shifting lines between health and illness.

Forgiveness
June 1997

I turned to my husband and asked in a tearful voice, "How can I leave?" We were standing by my father's bed at New York University Hospital. At seventy-nine, he was an aging man with Alzheimer's disease, but it was a virus that had brought him to the hospital. He had improved physically since his admission, but his mental deterioration had accelerated.

My relationship to my father had shifted in the last few years, as his dementia had become more pronounced. Alzheimer's had silenced his powerful verbal abuse. His lambasting insults, a sharp contrast to his occasional tender remarks, were in the past. The years had helped me come to terms with him and our relationship. Now we had quiet times together when we looked at art books or at photos of his grandchildren. Painful memories of my childhood and adolescent years had given way to feelings of compassion for a life interrupted and unfulfilled.

My husband and I had driven down from Boston. When we had first entered the hospital room, I had walked right past my father's bed, past the curtain separating him from his neighbor, and found myself staring at a young man talking on the telephone. Turning around, I had moved back to the first bed and looked at a stranger.

"Is this my father?" I asked, of no one in particular. The nurse adjusting his I.V. looked up.

Asking and answering my question in the same breath, I said, "Is that William Snyder? I'm his daughter. It is, isn't it?"

"Yes, dear," replied the nurse. "We're adjusting his medication. It will be a few minutes." The nurse drew the curtain around my father's bed.

Putting his arm around me, my husband asked, "Are you okay?"

"I just can't believe that's him. I knew this would be tough, but…" My voice trailed off. I was remembering my grandmother, my father's mother, as I last saw her in a nursing home. The shock of seeing my father in a hospital, for the first time in my life, had stunned me. His unshaven face and the tens of pounds of weight loss had combined to make him unrecognizable.

After the nurse had completed her work and drawn back the curtain and revealed me, I had seen a momentary glimmer of recognition in my father's eyes and then watched it disappear into a vast unknown. I had spent the next hour going through the photo album I had created for him, turning the pages and naming for him the people in the pictures. Then we had sat in silence. How could I leave him?

"Maybe there's something you want to say to him before we go," my husband said. "I'll just be out in the sun room." He squeezed my hand and left the room.

I thought that I didn't really have anything to say, maybe "I love you." That was something I had been feeling increasingly since his illness, an amorphous emotion that had often been lost in my connection to this charming but difficult, this loving but alcoholic and emotionally abusive man.

Then it occurred to me. I remembered some words about forgiveness that I had recently heard: To forgive is not to condone but to let go of one's resentments and to heal. His illness had brought me closer to this moment.

I looked at my father, who seemed to be puzzled now, as though he in his way was trying to work out our relationship. I looked into his blue eyes (my inheritance) and said, "Dad, I forgive you.... I love you." My voice was choked with emotion and somehow my father responded to this. His face scrunched up with concern, and he exclaimed, "What, where, hey?"

I kissed my hand and placed it on his cheek. Already, his eyes were staring off into the distance. "I forgive you," I repeated softly.

Perhaps I then said good-bye. I don't remember. Maybe I said "See ya," because "Good-bye" had a finality that I wasn't ready for.

I walked out into the corridor, down the hall, and into the sun room, where large windows faced the East River. A patient and a few visitors were talking with one another there. My husband was looking out at the water. I crossed the room to where he was standing, put my arms around him, and said, "Thank you. I think he heard me."

When Death Knocks at the Door
April 2005

We don't do death well in this culture. We recoil from discussions about death because we feel so deeply. Death triggers old losses, which we've not fully mourned. We fear our own demise, our absence, our nothingness. If we don't speak of death or loss, maybe it can't come into our lives. But then when it does, we are so unprepared.

But death came knocking at our door recently. The struggles of Terry Schiavo and Pope John Paul II forced each of us to think about the end of our lives, even while we shuddered at such thoughts. My friend Martha told me that living wills and dying became dinner table conversation for her family. She, her husband, and her sons pondered what they would want if they were in a vegetative state, what constituted life for each of them.

Last Thursday, I stared at the client form where I had to comment on a scheduled session that never happened. I placed a check on the line marked "cancellation," but that was a lie. I stared at the blank page again, unwilling to write that my client was dead after routine surgery, for then I would have to accept the fact. It was too stark, shocking, sad, unexpected. I finally wrote "client deceased."

That same day, the Vatican announced that the Pope would not enter a hospital for further medical treatment for Parkinson's disease. I was relieved that he had heeded his own words from 1998 that keeping patients alive by "extraordinary or disproportionate means" went against the principles of Catholicism. I was surprised that a lump formed in my throat and tears came to my eyes when I heard of the Pope's death on

Saturday. I didn't think that I was crying for the Pope, but for my client and for the fighting over Terry Schiavo's life that we had just witnessed. And for the losses that death triggers in each of us. I quietly wondered if there were deep feelings that Terry Schiavo's parents had been trying to avoid by keeping her alive.

When I learned that this Pope, who inspired the Solidarity movement and condemned capital punishment and the war in Iraq, was also the first to attend services in a synagogue, I knew that despite my distaste for his social conservatism, there was much to mourn, and tears came to my eyes again.

Soon, I thought of death closer to my heart. I remembered my father, who, in 1996 after ten years of Alzheimer's disease, was hospitalized with pneumonia. He recovered after a few weeks, but it was clear that my mother could no longer care for him at home. He entered a nursing home, where he lived for two more years. He hadn't signed a living will nor did I know what my mother's wishes were then. My siblings and I agreed that our father would only want end-of-life measures to keep him comfortable. He had lost his ability to formulate words and could no longer recognize faces. He had no control over his bladder and bowels. I remember when I visited him in the nursing home six weeks before he died. I sat with him for twenty minutes. He stared into space, made some sounds. I had brought in one of his art books to capture his interest. The art, once his passion, seemed to mean nothing to him. But he suddenly looked at me, smiled, and said, "You are beautiful." I was stunned. Did I believe my father's aphasia had disappeared? Maybe for those few seconds. But was that enough? His momentary lucidity vanished into vacancy and I never saw that man again. He died when he forgot how to eat.

When my father developed Alzheimer's disease, he quickly lost his ability to formulate words. Towards the end of his life, he was only present in the here and now. When he was still eating, he might appreciate a bite of salmon but would then forget to continue with his meal. I pondered the quality of life. An opinionated man, his personality had disappeared with his words. But wasn't there value in a moment-to-moment existence?

Songwriter Bob Franke underlines the dark permanence of death: "For the hole in the middle of a pretty good life, I only face it 'cause it's here to stay, not my father nor my mother nor my daughter nor my lover nor the highway made it go away."

It's true. The deep feelings never do go away.

My Journey with Barbara Jordan
January 1996

I remember Barbara Jordan from my adolescence as I, along with much of the nation, was riveted to the television by the Watergate impeachment hearings. I was eighteen years old in 1974. She was a big part of what drew me to the Watergate enigma.

The mystery of politics mattered, but Jordan's voice shone above those men with whom she presided. Her oratory and her shining black skin captured me during a time when I was coming of age, learning what black and white meant, learning what right and wrong meant.

And then after all the hearings, after President Nixon resigned, I lost track of her, though I knew she remained a vibrant personality on the political scene.

I continued my studies at Goucher College, then a women's college, where women like Barbara Jordan were our role models — visionaries such as Emma Goldman, Gertrude Stein, May Sarton, Ann Sexton, Gloria Steinem.

But where Ms. Jordan went in my world, I did not know. When I continued on my journey and taught high school history, other women became the central figures. It was not for some time after I was diagnosed with multiple sclerosis, in 1981, that I learned that Ms. Jordan also had MS. That larger-than-life figure whom I had held as an idol, she, too, had that illness of mystery and cruelty. I would again have her as a role model. She used a wheelchair now and continued her career as a teacher and scholar.

And then, on the news this morning I hear that Barbara Jordan has died, at the age of fifty-nine. "No," I shout out, "it can't be, God please, don't say it was from MS. People don't die of multiple sclerosis." Later in the day, I hear that her death was from complications of leukemia. Why did such a woman, who gave so much, get hit with the unfairness of two illnesses?

I happen to be having an exacerbation of MS on this day. I've had scotomas, or areas of diminished vision, in both eyes for several days; when I look to the right, there is nothing in my visual field. MS is still here. And I am here. My day is a tough one. I sit in fear and anger. I pray. Did you ever do this, Barbara? It is people like you to whom I pray, to spirits like yours from whom I ask for the gifts of patience, hope, and faith. It is people like you who offer us all a belief in the best of ourselves. God bless you and good-bye.

About the Author

Dana Snyder-Grant, LICSW, is a writer and a clinical social worker, specializing in chronic illness and disability. She is a columnist for her local newspaper in Acton, Massachusetts, where she lives in a cohousing community with her husband and two cats.

Dana can be reached at danasg@newview.org or you can learn more about Dana and her work at http://www.snyder-grant.org/dana.

CPSIA information can be obtained
at www.ICGtesting.com
Printed in the USA
LVOW11s1514020317
525947LV00001B/177/P